BRAIDS, BUNCHES & PIGTAILS FOR GIRLS

This book is dedicated to
my number one fans
my sweet Magnolia and Indy 'Nay Nay'.
Mama loves you.

Published by Apple Press in 2016

Apple Press
74-77 White Lion Street
London N1 9PF
UK
www.apple-press.com

Falkirk Council		
Askews & Holts	2016	
646.724	£12.99	

10 9 8 7 6 5 4 3 2 1

Manufactured in China

ISBN: 978-1-84543-641-4

Publisher: Mark Searle
Editorial Director: Isheeta Mustafi
Commissioning Editor: Alison Morris
Editor: Erin Chamberlain
Junior Editor: Abbie Sharman
Art Director: Michelle Rowlandson
Design concept: Agata Rybicka
Layout: Kate Haynes
Illustrations: Sarah Skeate

Image credits
Front cover (clockwise from top): hair Jenny
Strebe; photography Sarah Bishop; models
Htoorahmu Pee, Eliana Brown, Kendall Peck.

Back cover (right to left): hair Jenny Strebe;
photography Sarah Bishop; model
Magnolia Strebe.

BRAIDS, BUNCHES & PIGTAILS FOR GIRLS

50 fun and easy hair dos for school,
parties and playdates

JENNY STREBE

APPLE

Contents

CHAPTER ONE

Ponytails

CHAPTER TWO

Braids

CHAPTER THREE

Pigtails

CHAPTER FOUR

Buns and Twists

Introduction

As a professional hairstylist and educational director for more than 15 years, I have cut, styled and coloured hair of every type and texture. Dividing my time between Arizona, Los Angeles and New York, my hair artistry has been seen on TV and video, in high fashion publications and on the fashion catwalk. My real passion lies in empowering women and inspiring confidence with great hair and I do this every day on my blog, Confessions of a Hairstylist. In just three years, it's become the go-to for hair how-to's, with more than three million views on YouTube™.

Away from the glamour of the salon, I'm also a dedicated mum of two. I know how challenging it can be to keep your child's hair not only looking chic and cool but also neat and practical for school. That's why I developed this book. I have designed 50 individual hair looks from traditional updos with a modern twist to sensible styles for everyday. Whether it's a formal look for a family wedding or a fun stage style for your child's next performance, this book has a hairdo to suit every occasion.

My step-by-step instructions are accompanied by detailed illustrations, so it's really easy to follow and will help to overcome any challenges you have with your child's hair. We've simplified each technique and included a few of my industry secrets along the way so you can perfect the look quickly, with minimal protest. Even if your child doesn't have the perfect hair for a particular style, my pro tips for each look will help you to achieve it. This book will give you the confidence and the know-how to achieve any style or look on your child.

There's never a bad hair day with this book by your side.

Jenny Strebe

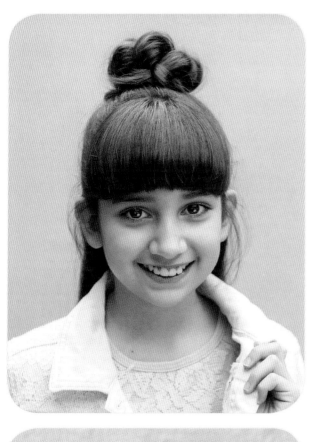
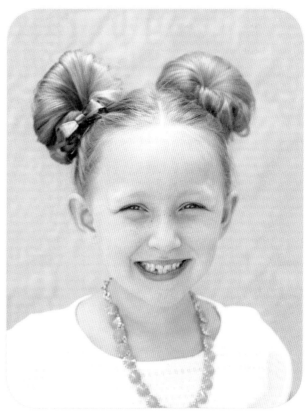
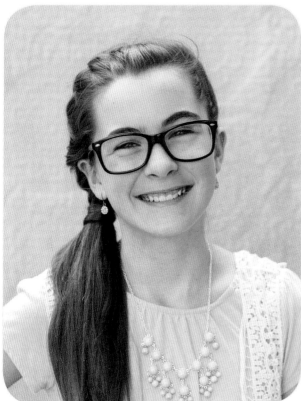
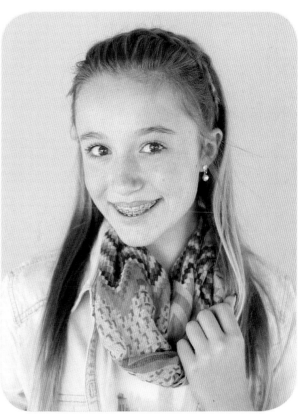

Getting Started

The trick to styling your child's hair is all in the tools. Just like adults, every child's hair is different, and how you style each hair type is also varied. There are several accessories and hair tools that can help make your child's hair more manageable when styling. Helping your child look good will make them feel good too and their confidence will shine through. The following tools are a big part of taking care of your child's hair, and will help you achieve some of the looks in this book.

Tools

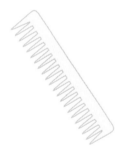

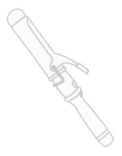

WIDE-TOOTHED COMB
This is a hair care must-have. A wide-toothed comb is preferable to tighter combs because it doesn't pull on the hair, causing it to break. The wide teeth allow the hair to glide through the comb and remove unwanted knots simply and painlessly.

CURLING TONGS
Some of the hairstyles in this book require this styling tool. Always be careful when using it around your child because it works by applying heat to help create waves and curls in the hair. The clamp allows you to hold on to the hair as you ease it through the hair tongs. Many curling tongs have an adjustable heat setting to suit all different hair types.

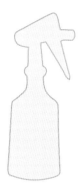
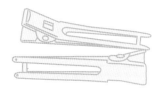
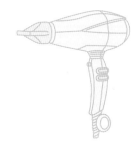

WATER SPRAY BOTTLE

This is an essential for taming flyaways, fine hair and newly washed hair that is too soft to style. A simple spray of water will give the hair some grip without using nasty chemicals, and allow you to style it more easily.

DUCK-BILL CLIPS

These are great for keeping hair in place or out of your child's face during styling, especially if they have a fringe or layers.

HAIRDRYER

Most of the hairstyles we feature in the book can be styled while the hair is wet, but sometimes you will need to dry the hair first. A hairdryer will also help to give it some volume, if needed.

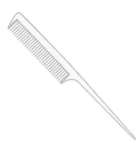
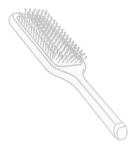

RAT TAIL COMB

Also known as a weaving comb or tail comb. This type of comb has a fine-toothed side and a narrow end made of plastic or metal. This comb is great for dividing the hair into sections and creating partings.

DETANGLING BRUSH

This is, without a doubt, the best way to brush a child's hair without pulling, tugging, breaking or hurting their scalp in the process. This invention has saved many mums' (and children's) lives because it means less fussing and more styling. There are a few different brands so find the one that suits you.

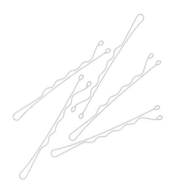
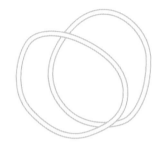
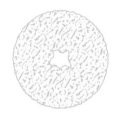

BOBBY PINS

These hairpins, also known as hair grips or kirby grips, are essential for holding an elaborate hairstyle in place. They are great for controlling layered hair and pinning it into place for long periods. Bobby pins are also a great way to keep a fringe out of your child's face when they're in the growing-out phase.

HAIR ELASTICS

These are essential for styling to hold the hair in place. They are the most practical hair accessory, and perfect for casual hairstyling. You can opt for a scrunchie if you prefer a natural ponytail with a touch of style and difference.

SOCK-BUN DOUGHNUT

If you want a quick and easy hairstyle that keeps the hair up and out of the way but still looks super chic, the simple sock-bun doughnut is your go-to accessory. It makes beautiful hair buns in less than a minute. It is also super lightweight, so it won't hurt your child's scalp if left in for long periods. It will keep it tight and in place for hours.

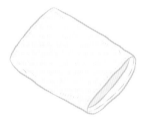
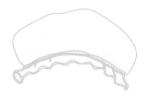

SILK PILLOWCASE

This is optional but will definitely keep your child's hair healthy, silky and smooth, minimising breakage and messy bedhead. It's also a natural and breathable fabric for your child to sleep on.

SATIN BONNET

This helps to protect the hair and maintain moisture while your child sleeps, and minimise frizz. It's also great for maintaining the natural state of the hair for a more relaxed look.

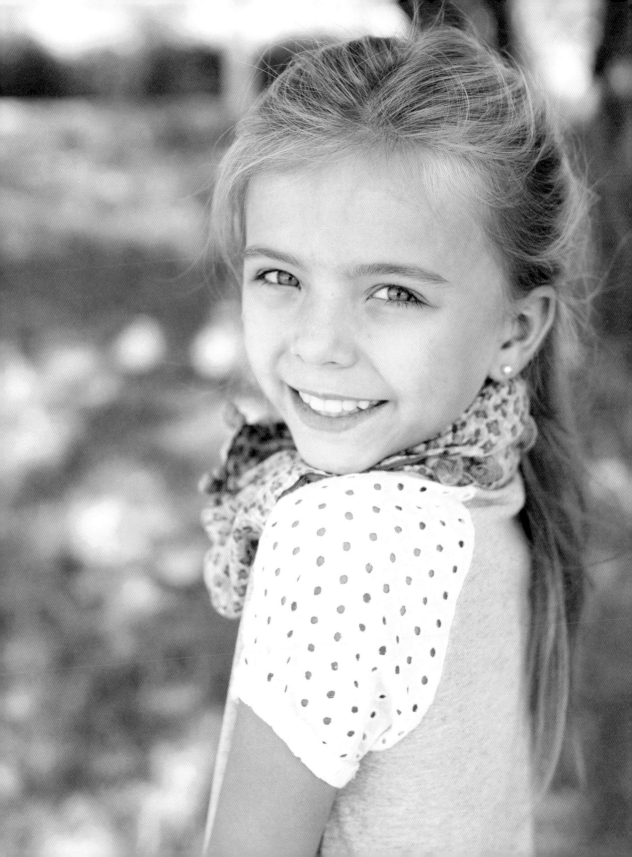

Hair Care

Healthy hair starts here! Not taking care of your child's hair can lead to lacklustre locks. Implementing a few common care practises into your routine is all it takes to keep your child's hair looking shiny and fresh. Here are a few basic steps that will help you to care for their hair, from how to shampoo it properly to how many products you really need. Not only will it prevent damaged hair, but it will also make it easier to work with when styling. Incorporating these techniques into your daily routine will also help your child develop healthy hair-care habits from an early age.

HOW TO WASH YOUR CHILD'S HAIR

It's important you wet the hair and the scalp with warm water before applying shampoo. Once wet, rub the shampoo really well into the hair and massage the scalp to stimulate the hair follicles. This will remove any debris or oil at the roots. Try not to over-wash – just two to three times a week should be enough. Over-washing will lead to flyaways. Use a shampoo and conditioner created for your little one's hair texture. Choose something that's free from nasty chemicals too, as the scalp is one of the most absorbent parts of your body. When shampooing, teach your child how to massage their scalp and wash from the top of the head downwards. Rinse well with warm water until the soap suds have completely gone. When you dry your child's hair, wrap it up into a towel and just squeeze it dry. Don't vigorously rub the hair or you will damage it and cause it to break.

USE LEAVE-IN CONDITIONER

If your child has frizzy or flyaway-prone hair, use a leave-in conditioner to tame it. Purchase one in a spray bottle so you can apply it directly to the hair. There are plenty of child-friendly products available – look for a brand that works for you and your child's hair type. Use leave-in conditioner on wet or dry hair, but for taming flyaways it's best to spray it on the hair while it's damp. Leave-in conditioner is great to apply to hair to minimise any pain when removing knots or tangles, and for helping to style clean hair.

WHY YOU NEED TO BRUSH

Brushing is really important to maintain healthy hair. It helps to stimulate the scalp and encourage the hair to grow. It also distributes the natural oils from the roots to the ends, which prevents dryness and is a great way to keep hair shiny without using products. Source a brush with soft and pliable bristles that's designed for tackling tangles. Don't brush your child's hair when it is wet as this can damage the hair and cause split ends. If you have to brush it when wet, use a wide-toothed comb. It's much gentler and your child will thank you for it.

LET IT AIR DRY

Most of the braids in this book can be achieved with wet hair. In fact, this is the best way to style a braid without the hassle of soft, slippery, dry hair that can be difficult to work with. Once you have braided the hair when wet, just let it air dry – there is no need for any sprays or products. You can use a spray bottle filled with water to soften any stray hairs.

DOES YOUR CHILD HAVE FINE HAIR?

Fine hair tends to be more oily, which means you might need to wash it more often; alternatively, you could use a dry shampoo to make it last longer in between shampoos. Dry shampoo is also great for creating bulk; this is especially handy when you need to pancake braids – stretching the braids out a bit so they appear thicker. You can even curl fine hair prior to styling to achieve a fuller look.

DOES YOUR CHILD HAVE THICK HAIR?

When washing thick hair, pay attention to the roots. Since there is so much more hair, it will require some extra scrubbing at the roots and a thorough rinse. Sometimes thick hair won't rinse all the way, so be sure to rinse until the water is free from suds.

DOES YOUR CHILD HAVE FRIZZY HAIR?

Choose a shampoo and conditioner that's specific to frizzy hair. It will help smooth and control the hair so it's ready for styling. Always scrunch or lightly towel dry the hair when wet; don't vigorously brush it or you will end up with very frizzy hair, very quickly. Always use a wide-toothed comb to detangle it when wet. You can even use a frizz control serum before drying to tame it even further and ready it for styling.

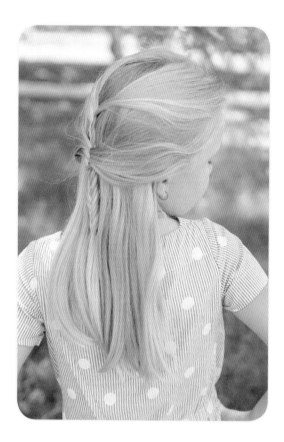

HOW TO STYLE YOUR CHILD'S HAIR NATURALLY

If you don't want to use commercial hairsprays and products on your child's hair, then there are gentler, more natural ways to tame it during styling. You can purchase an inexpensive spray bottle from your local store and fill it with water. This is a great alternative to products because a simple spray of water on the hair can provide much-needed grip when fashioning an updo. It's also a great finishing spray for flattening any flyaways. If you want to add some natural shine, put a few drops of organic cold-pressed coconut oil into the water. This is great for maintaining the health of the hair too. Some hairdos may need to be dampened slightly before styling, so always have a spray bottle nearby.

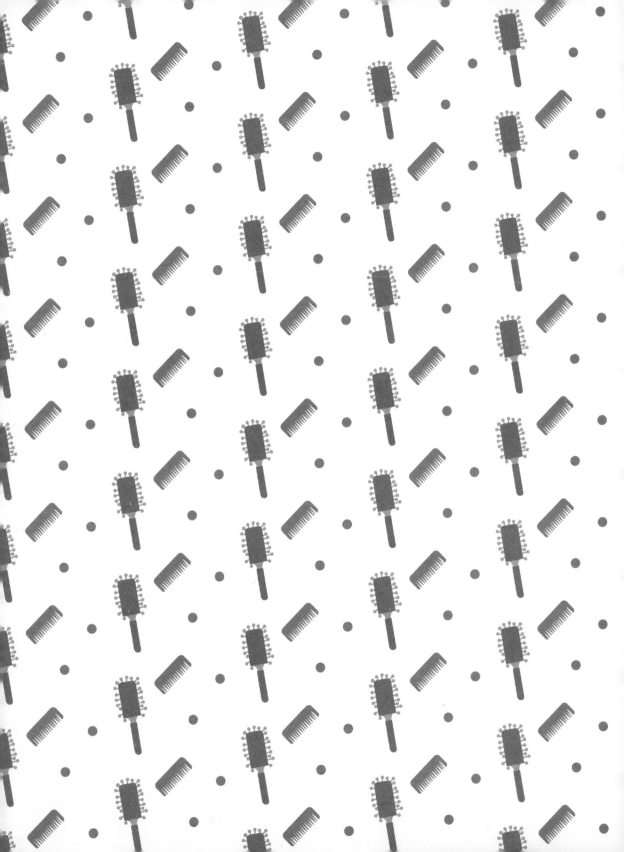

CHAPTER ONE

Ponytails

High Crown Ponytail

This is probably the number one go-to hairdo for mums for its classic look and simplicity. The high crown ponytail always looks good, and while you might think you know how it's done, there is an art to getting it right. It works well with all hair types; however, fine- to medium-textured hair is best, as it will not weigh your ponytail down. The style is suited to straight and wavy textured hair, but, as always, feel free to experiment with your child's hair, whatever the type or texture. Be sure to fasten it tightly with an elastic or you may end up redoing it throughout the day. Thankfully it's a fairly easy style to replicate!

DIFFICULTY LEVEL
Easy

IDEAL HAIR
Medium to long; fine to medium texture; straight to wavy

ACCESSORIES
A pretty ribbon looks great tied around the elastic.

SEE ALSO
High Pigtails, page 78

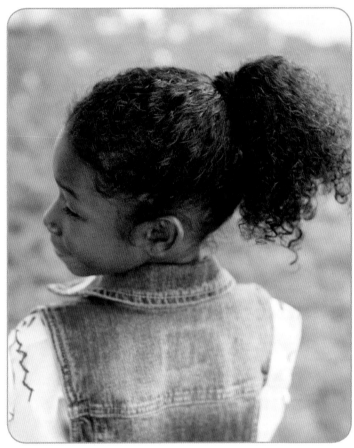

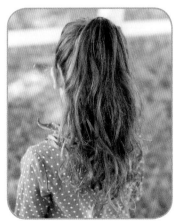

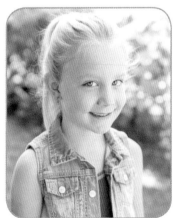

Get the look

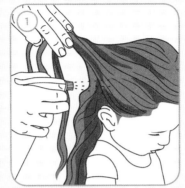
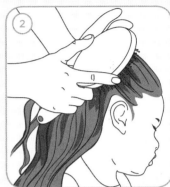

WHAT YOU NEED

- Brush or comb
- Water spray bottle
- Hair elastic
- Bobby pin
- Flexible-hold hairspray

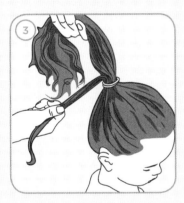
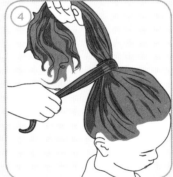
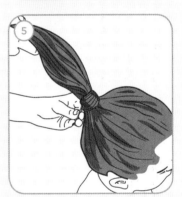

1. Brush or comb the hair until it is smooth and free from tangles. Lightly mist the hair with the water spray and then comb straight back to the crown of the head.

2. Gather the hair together into your other hand. Hold tight to create a high ponytail. Secure in place with an elastic.

3. Take a small section of hair from the underside of the ponytail.

4. Wrap the section of hair around the base of the ponytail to cover the elastic. Attach a bobby pin to the end of that section of hair.

5. Push the bobby pin into the ponytail to secure into place. Lightly mist with a flexible-hold hairspray to set the look.

TOP TIP

If the hair is flyaway prone, add a tiny bit of gel to the water in the spray bottle for extra hold and to ensure flyways don't fall out of your ponytail.

Half Ponytail

This simple way to get a child's hair out of her face is easy to create, but it does not have to look basic. Secure a small piece of hair around the elastic to create a seamless look from the back and add a touch of high fashion to an everyday hairstyle. It's the perfect 'do for school, playdates, parties and casual gatherings.

DIFFICULTY LEVEL
Easy

IDEAL HAIR
Medium to long; straight to wavy

ACCESSORIES
Fix a fashionable headband or decorative clips at the front of the hair to keep flyaways at bay.

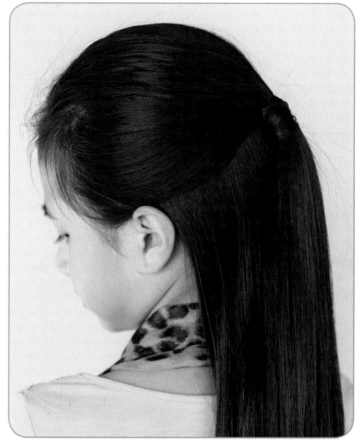

 SEE ALSO
Side Twists,
page 98

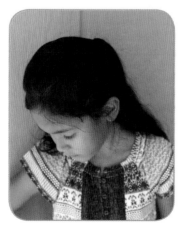

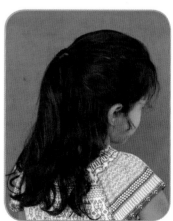

Get the look

WHAT YOU NEED

- Brush or comb
- Hair elastic
- Bobby pin

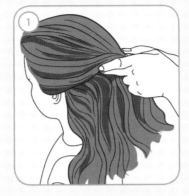

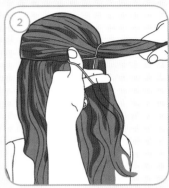

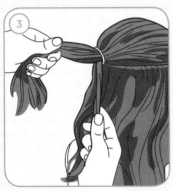

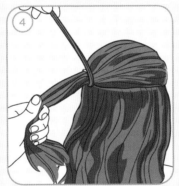

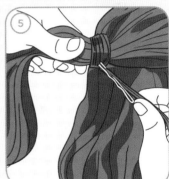

1. Brush or comb the hair until it is smooth and free from tangles. Split hair in half from the top to the bottom.

2. Gather the hair in the top half and create a half ponytail. Secure in place with an elastic.

3. Take a small section of hair from the underside of the ponytail.

4. Wrap the hair around the elastic.

5. Attach a bobby pin to the end of that section of hair. Push the bobby pin into the ponytail to secure into place.

TOP TIP

If the hair is silky or prone to flyaways, create this style on damp hair to easily grip the hair and smooth frizzes.

Ropebraid Ponytail

This polished pony is a sleek look from front to back. It is a clever way to secure baby hair or flyaways too. It might look tricky, but once you understand how the braid works, it is actually easy to create. This unique update on the ponytail is a fun and fashionable style for school, birthday parties and playdates. It is also a chic option for formal events.

DIFFICULTY LEVEL
Medium

IDEAL HAIR
Long; fine to medium texture; straight to wavy

ACCESSORIES
A large bow, headband or hair scarf will add interest to the hairline.

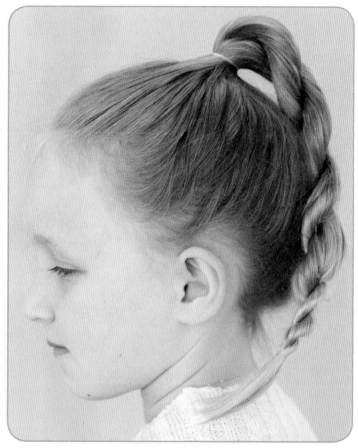

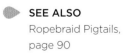 **SEE ALSO**
Ropebraid Pigtails,
page 90

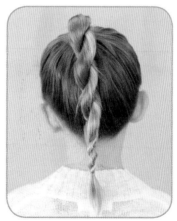

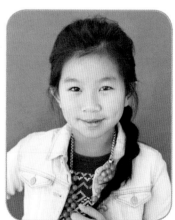

Get the look

WHAT YOU NEED

- Brush or comb
- Water spray bottle
- Hair elastics

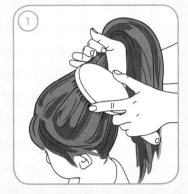

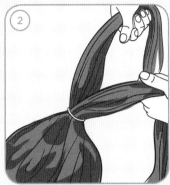

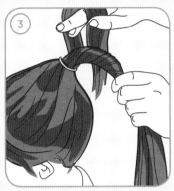

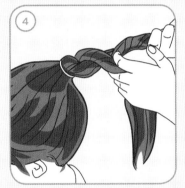

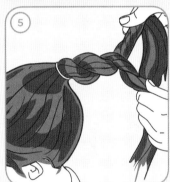

1. Brush or comb the hair until it is smooth and free from tangles. Lightly mist the hair with the water spray and brush straight back to the crown of the head to create a high ponytail. Secure in place with an elastic.

2. Divide the hair inside the ponytail into two equal parts.

3. Take each of the two sections and twist them clockwise.

4. Pass the left-hand section under the right-hand section while keeping the hair in each section securely twisted.

5. Continue this technique until you reach the ends of the hair. Secure in place with an elastic.

TOP TIP

If the hair has layers, add a bit of curl to the hair prior to starting the ropebraid ponytail. This will ensure that the layers will blend into the ponytail, instead of sticking out.

Pageant Ponytail

If you have a big event or a special occasion planned, this formal version of the standard ponytail is the perfect hairstyle. It is full of volume with soft curls that spill effortlessly from the back, and the front features a chic pompadour. This elegant look is amazing on younger children with its messy vibe that is not overly styled or stuffy. Create this look for weddings, anniversaries, dance recitals and performances.

DIFFICULTY LEVEL
Hard

IDEAL HAIR
Medium to long; fine to thick texture; wavy to curly

ACCESSORIES
A sparkly headband or clips fixed where the pompadour meets the ponytail will look great.

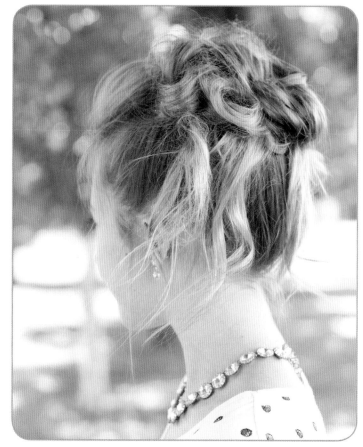

 SEE ALSO
Ballerina Bun,
page 114

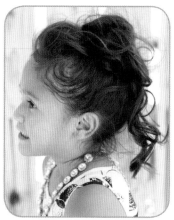
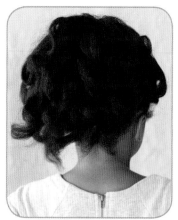

Get the look

WHAT YOU NEED

- Brush or comb
- Hair clip
- Hair elastic
- Bobby pins
- Medium-hold hairspray
- 2.5-cm (1-inch) curling tongs

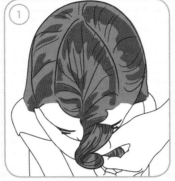

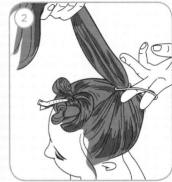

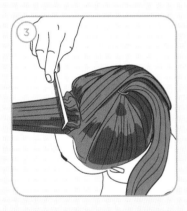

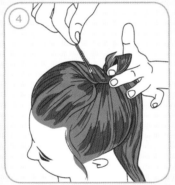

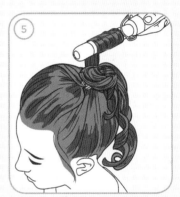

1. Brush or comb the hair. Take a small triangle section of hair from the crown to the forehead and clip away.

2. Create a high ponytail with the remaining hair. Secure in place with an elastic.

3. Unclip the hair inside the triangle. Split it into two sections and tease it by running a comb down the length of the hair to the roots at the hairline.

4. Brush the triangle section back to the top of the ponytail. Twist the section near the elastic and secure in place with bobby pins.

5. Curl the ponytail, taking 2.5-cm (1-inch) sections of hair, spritzing each one with hairspray and curling with 2.5-cm (1-inch) curling tongs. Gently brush the hair out, then twist each section and bobby pin it into place so all the tendrils don't hang down.

TOP TIP

If the hair doesn't hold curls, use smaller-sized curling tongs. This will create tighter curls so that when the curl drops, the hair will still have some body.

Double Braided Ponytail

A quick and simple way to wear a ponytail. If your child feels the heat, it is great for the summer months to keep the hair off her neck, but it's also a pretty ponytail all year round. This style works well on medium to thick hair that is straight to wavy in texture because it helps to define the braid. However, it can look great on curly hair, so don't hesitate to give it a try even though your child's hair texture may be a little different.

DIFFICULTY LEVEL
Easy

IDEAL HAIR
Medium to long; medium to thick texture; straight to wavy

ACCESSORIES
Embellish this look with a bow at the base of the ponytail.

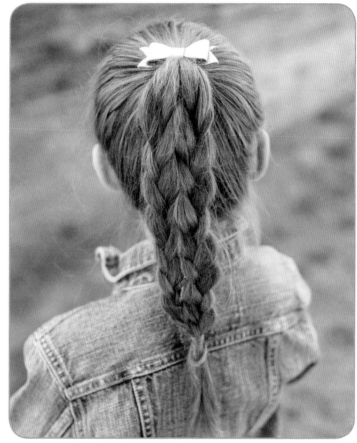

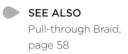 **SEE ALSO**
Pull-through Braid,
page 58

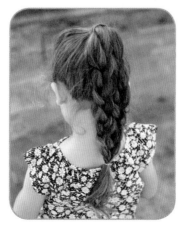

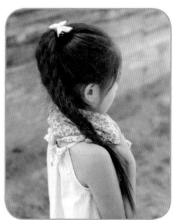

Get the look

WHAT YOU NEED
- Brush or comb
- Hair elastics
- Bobby pin

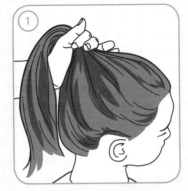
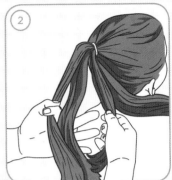
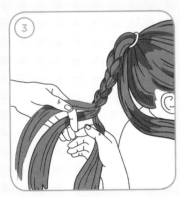
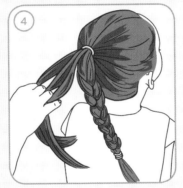
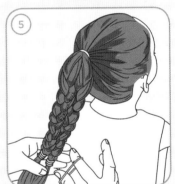

1. Brush or comb the hair until it is smooth and free from tangles. Gather it into a high ponytail at the crown. Secure in place with an elastic.
2. Divide the hair in the ponytail in half. Split one section of the hair into three equal sections.
3. Braid one section of the hair. Take the section from the right up and over to the middle and then take the section from the left up and over to the middle. Repeat, right following left, until you reach the ends of the hair. Secure in place with an elastic.
4. Braid the other half of the ponytail.
5. Interlock the braided sections, holding the braids together and weaving a bobby pin, held vertically, up and down mid-braid. Secure the ends of the two braids together with an elastic.

TOP TIP

If the hair is fine, make the braids appear full by pulling on hair from each side of the braid.

Messy Low Ponytail

When you're short on time, you need a low-fuss hairstyle that's high on style. This low ponytail is a winner for mums with fussy little ones who don't want to sit still for long periods, but the end result is as snazzy as the more intricate styles. This fashionable update on the beloved low pony is suited to casual playdates, school days and catch-ups with friends.

DIFFICULTY LEVEL
Easy

IDEAL HAIR
Medium to long; fine to thick texture; wavy to curly

ACCESSORIES
A headband or scarf wrapped around the head makes this look really special.

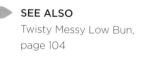 **SEE ALSO**
Twisty Messy Low Bun,
page 104

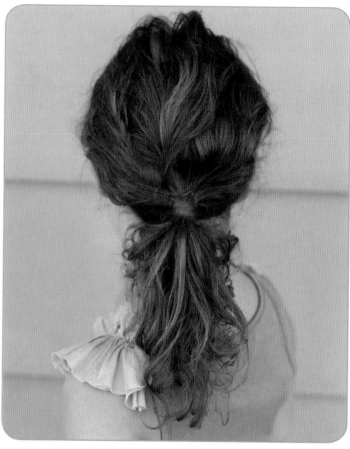

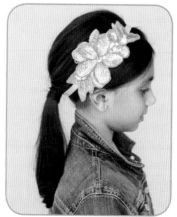

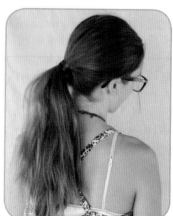

Get the look

WHAT YOU NEED

- Brush or comb
- Hair elastic
- Bobby pin

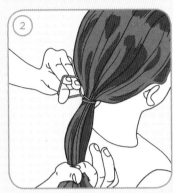
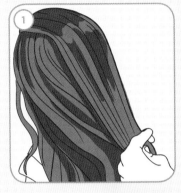
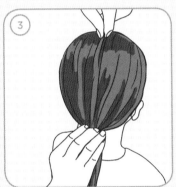
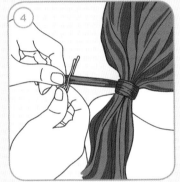
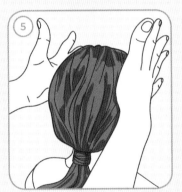

1. Brush or comb the hair until it is smooth and free from tangles. Lightly finger brush the hair towards the nape of the neck.

2. Gather the hair into a loose low ponytail. Secure in place with an elastic.

3. Deliberately create a messy finish where the hair covers the scalp in the ponytail. Hold the base of the elastic while pulling strands of hair above the elastic upwards.

4. Take a small section of hair from the underside of the ponytail. Wrap the section of hair around the base of the ponytail to cover the elastic. Attach a bobby pin to the end of that section of hair and push the bobby pin into the ponytail to secure into place.

5. To finish, take the palms of your hands and rub them along the sides of the hairline to deliberately form flyaways.

TOP TIP

If the hair is straight, curl the hair with 2.5-cm (1-inch) curling tongs prior to pulling it into the ponytail. This will create volume and allow you to get a messier texture.

Pretty Party Ponytail

When it's time to celebrate, this spunky take on the typical ponytail is party approved. Pump up the volume with this high version that's practical, pretty and easy. Your little girl can dance and twirl without a care in the world because once this style is set you can forget about it – it won't budge.

DIFFICULTY LEVEL
Easy

IDEAL HAIR
Medium to long; minimal layers; straight to wavy

ACCESSORIES
Fix some fancy clips along the hairline for a fun party look.

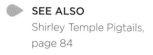 **SEE ALSO**
Shirley Temple Pigtails, page 84

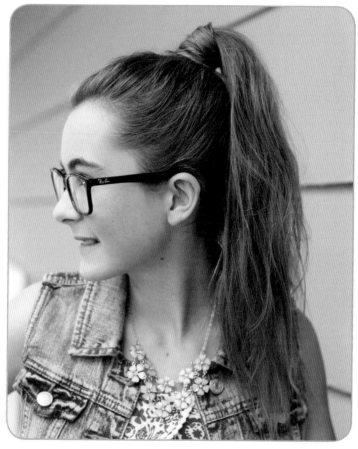

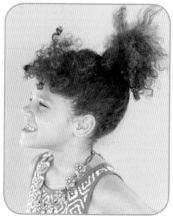

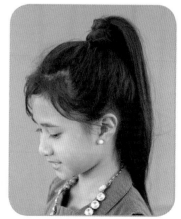

Get the look

WHAT YOU NEED

- Brush or comb
- Hair elastic
- Bobby pin

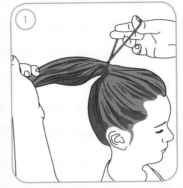

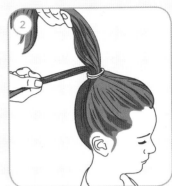

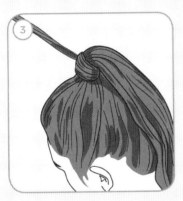

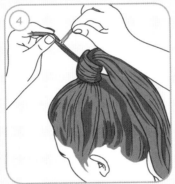

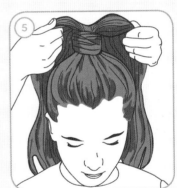

1. Brush or comb the hair until it is smooth and free from tangles. Gather it into a high ponytail at the top of the head. Secure in place with an elastic.

2. Take a large section of hair from the underside of the ponytail.

3. Wrap the section of hair around the elastic, wrapping upwards, away from the elastic and covering the ponytail, so that it extends the height of the ponytail from the head. Aim to achieve 2.5 to 5 cm (1 to 2 inches) of a 'sleeve' of hair as you wrap.

4. When you come to the end of the hair, attach a bobby pin to the end and secure the sleeve by placing the bobby pin into the opening of the elastic band and the wrapped hair.

5. Tighten the ponytail by dividing the hair in half and pulling it to the sides.

TOP TIP

If the hair is thick and won't easily stay up from the root, make the ponytail more secure by adding a couple more bobby pins along the sleeve of hair into the centre of the ponytail.

Viking Braid in Ponytail

Are you tired of the same old braid or ponytail? This style is the best of both worlds – it's a braid–pony fusion, based on a simple inside-out or reverse French braid, better known as a Dutch braid. If you already have some braiding skills, you will have no problems mastering this one. This braid is ideal for thick, straight hair as the more hair you have, the bigger the side Viking braid will be.

DIFFICULTY LEVEL
Medium

IDEAL HAIR
Medium to long; thick texture; straight

ACCESSORIES
Tie a pretty ribbon in a bow at the bottom of the braid to hide the elastic.

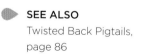

SEE ALSO
Twisted Back Pigtails, page 86

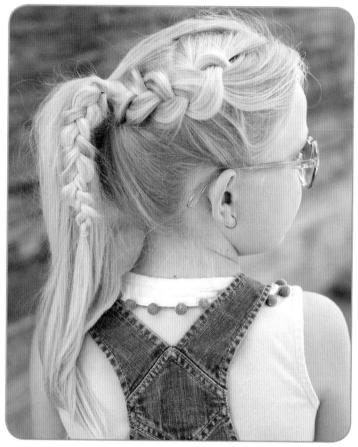

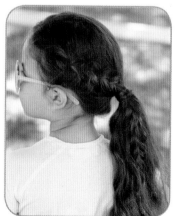

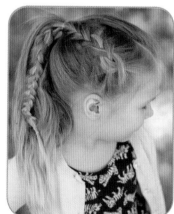

Get the look

WHAT YOU NEED

- Brush or comb
- Hair elastics

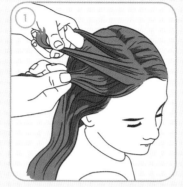

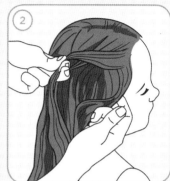

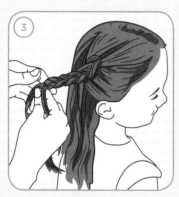

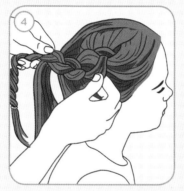

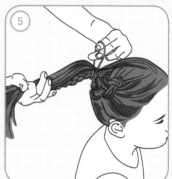

1. Brush or comb the hair. Make a centre parting and section out a small piece of hair from the front of the hairline. Divide it into three equal pieces.

2. Take the left section of hair under into the middle, taking the middle section to the left. Add hair from the hairline to the right section. Take the right section under into the middle. Add hair to the left section from the parting to the braid. Take the left section under into the middle. Repeat on the right side.

3. Braid to the ends, using the three-strand braiding technique (see page 25). Secure in place with an elastic.

4. Pancake the braid, pulling and stretching each side of the braid.

5. Gather the remaining hair into a high ponytail at the crown of the head. Add the braid and secure in place with an elastic.

TOP TIP

If the hair is silky and slippery, add sea salt spray before beginning to style. It will create texture and hold all day.

French Back Ponytail

This French braid meets ponytail hybrid combines two classic looks for one simple update on the traditional hairstyle. The front French braid gives the hair extra volume for a pretty pompadour effect, while the pony at the back keeps the look fresh and modern. It's another awesome school day hairdo but can be worn to any occasion, formal or casual, from weddings to birthday parties.

DIFFICULTY LEVEL
Easy

IDEAL HAIR
Long; medium to thick; straight to wavy

ACCESSORIES
Secure a cute bow or ribbon at the back.

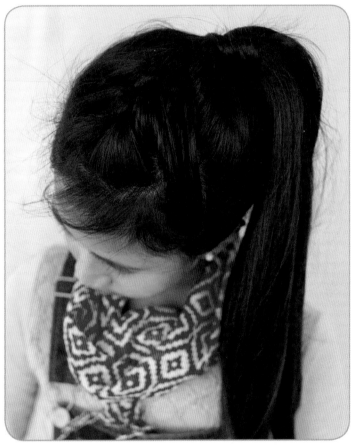

 SEE ALSO
Heart Braid,
page 68

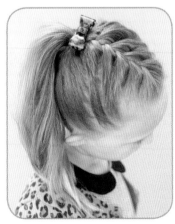

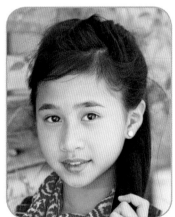

Get the look

WHAT YOU NEED

- Brush or comb
- Hair elastic

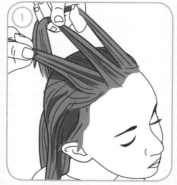
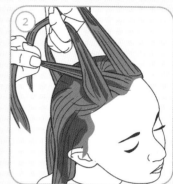
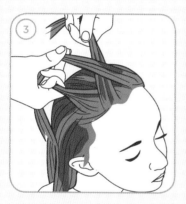
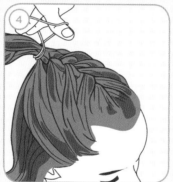
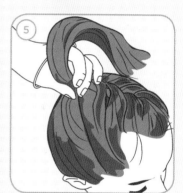

1. Brush or comb the hair. Section out a small piece of hair from the front of the hairline and divide it into three equal pieces.

2. Start a French braid (see page 44), starting with the right section. Take the right section and cross it over to the middle.

3. Cross the left section over to the middle. The section that started in the middle is now on the right, the right section is now on the left, and the left section moves to the middle.

4. Add hair from the hairline into the right section. Take it and the added hair to the middle. Repeat, adding hair to the sections on each side and moving right to left until you get to the crown of the head. Secure the base of the braid with an elastic.

5. Gather the remaining hair into a ponytail at the crown of the head, securing it where the braid finishes with another elastic.

TOP TIP

This is a great hairstyle for children growing out their fringe as the French braid will hold the shorter pieces of hair in place.

Braided Side Ponytail

A simple and stylish alternative to the regular ponytail, this fun style has a beautiful vibe your girl will love, and all her friends will too. It's polished enough for a formal event but the smart casual appeal also works for school, catch-ups with friends, family dinners and birthday parties.

DIFFICULTY LEVEL
Medium

IDEAL HAIR
Long; medium to thick; straight to wavy

ACCESSORIES
Elevate this stylish braid with a trendy headband or a big bow.

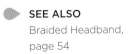 **SEE ALSO**
Braided Headband, page 54

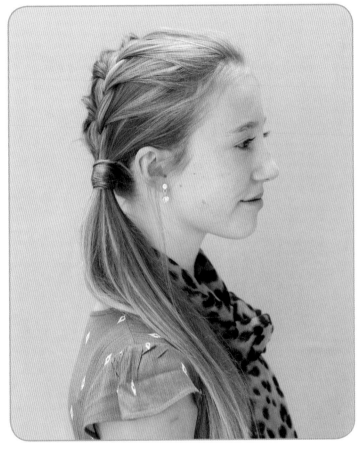

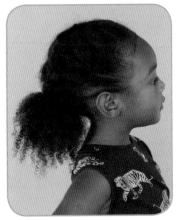

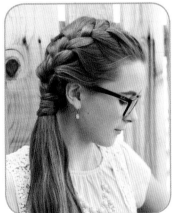

Get the look

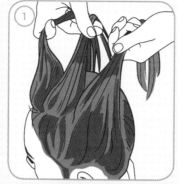
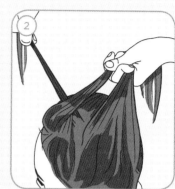

WHAT YOU NEED

- Brush or comb
- Hair elastic
- Bobby pin

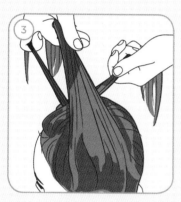
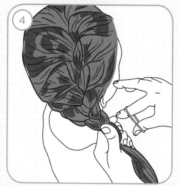
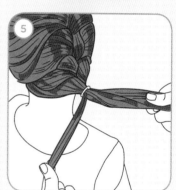

1. Brush or comb the hair. Brush the hair to one side and take a section from the hairline from the opposite side of the direction you want to braid. Divide into three equal sections.

2. Start a French braid (see page 44), braiding right then left. Add hair to each section, connecting the braid so that it moves across the head from the crown, behind the ear.

3. Continue to braid, moving left to right, adding hair to each section and taking it across to the middle.

4. Direct the braid to the opposite side of the head until you get to the nape of the neck. Secure into a side ponytail with an elastic.

5. To finish, take a small piece of hair from the underside of the ponytail and wrap it around the elastic, securing it with a bobby pin.

TOP TIP

If the hair is wavy or curly and prone to flyaways, add a bit of hair cream prior to braiding.

Lace Braid into Ponytail

The standard ponytail gets a stylish upgrade thanks to this sweet lace braid version. This style has a feminine feel with its elegant sweeping braid across the front of the hairline, but don't be fooled by its girly look because it's sturdy too. It will keep its shape all day, even withstanding rigorous play.

DIFFICULTY LEVEL
Easy

IDEAL HAIR
Long; fine to thick texture; minimal layers

ACCESSORIES
You can jazz it up with some pretty bows or trendy hair clips in bright colours.

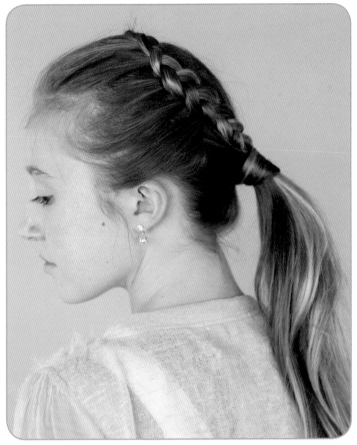

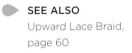 **SEE ALSO**
Upward Lace Braid,
page 60

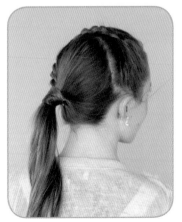

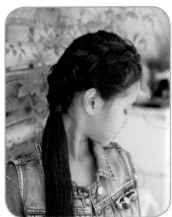

Get the look

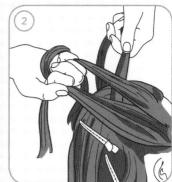
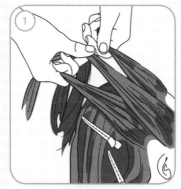
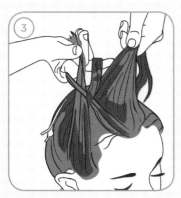
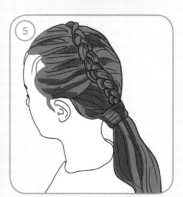
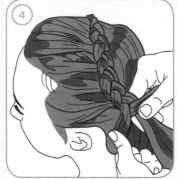

WHAT YOU NEED

- Brush or comb
- Hair clips
- Hair elastics
- Bobby pin

1. Brush or comb the hair. Take a section of hair from over the right ear. Clip away the rest. Divide the hair into three equal sections.

2. Take the right section and cross it under the middle section. Take the left section and cross it under the middle section. Continue to braid, adding hair to the right section only.

3. Direct the braid around the top of the head. When you reach the opposite ear, braid to the ends with the three-strand braid technique (see page 25). Secure the braid with an elastic.

4. Gather the unbraided hair and the braid and form a low ponytail, securing it with an elastic.

5. Wrap a small piece of hair from the underside of the ponytail around the elastic, and secure in place with a bobby pin. Remove the elastic from the end of the braid and unravel the hair up to the ponytail.

TOP TIP

Change the look of this style by where you choose to braid. If braided close to the hairline, the braid will stand out more. If braided further away, it won't make as much of a statement.

Topsy-tail Ponytail

Step up that ordinary ponytail style with some topsy-tail action. This chic take on the standard ponytail look is easy thanks to the amazing topsy-tail hair tool. Create something completely new in less than 30 seconds. That is music to any parent's ears! It is a fairly low-maintenance look, great for school or birthday parties.

DIFFICULTY LEVEL
Easy

IDEAL HAIR
Medium to long; baby fine to medium thickness; straight to wavy

ACCESSORIES
Use clips throughout the top of the hair for a dollop of fun!

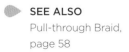 **SEE ALSO**
Pull-through Braid,
page 58

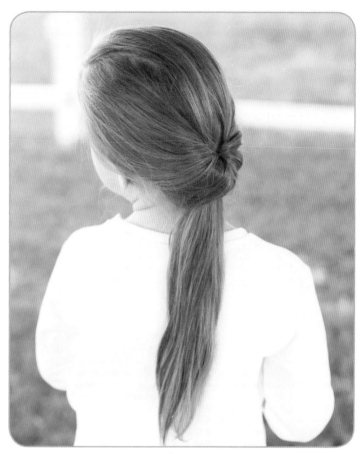

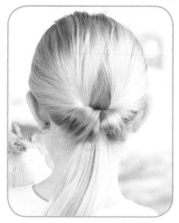

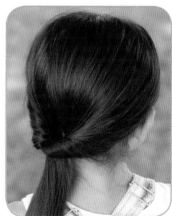

Get the look

WHAT YOU NEED

- Brush or comb
- Hair elastic
- Topsy-tail tool

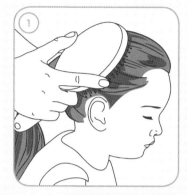

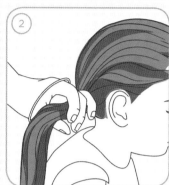

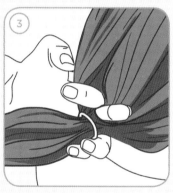

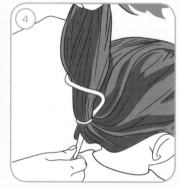

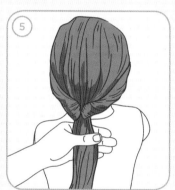

1. Brush or comb the hair until it is smooth and free from tangles. Brush all the hair to the nape of the neck.

2. Gather the hair into a loose low ponytail. Secure in place with an elastic.

3. Create a small gap behind the elastic and slide the pointy base of the topsy-tail tool in against the scalp of the head, pointing the tool down.

4. Thread the ponytail upwards through the loop of the topsy-tail.

5. Pull the topsy-tail down through the base of the ponytail, inverting the ponytail, creating your topsy-tail loop.

TOP TIP

If the topsy-tail ponytail is fuller on one side, even it out by gently pulling on each side of the twisted parts of the ponytail at the crown of the head to make it fuller.

Twisted Back Ponytail

If you're a fan of the pretty ponytail but ready to step it up to the next level, this is the style for you. The swirly details are a unique twist on the standard style but it's still simple to achieve. It's suited to thick textured hair because the twists will naturally look full. It's also great for taming naturally wavy or curly hair and the curls look great cascading from the back ponytail. You can play this up by curling them a little more with 3-cm (1¼-inch) curling tongs.

DIFFICULTY LEVEL
Easy

IDEAL HAIR
Long; medium to thick texture; straight or wavy

ACCESSORIES
A cute hair ribbon, coloured hair elastics or some hair clips will really give this style the wow factor.

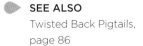

SEE ALSO
Twisted Back Pigtails, page 86

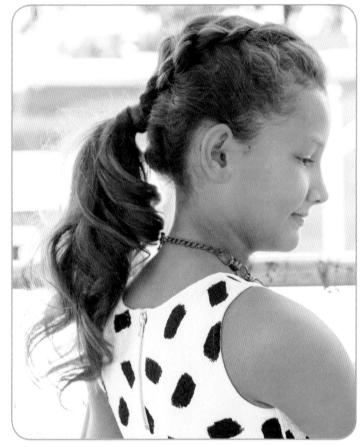

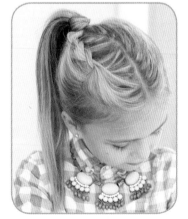

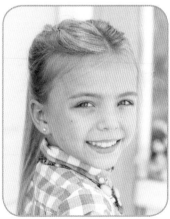

Get the look

WHAT YOU NEED

- Brush or comb
- Rat tail comb
- Hair elastics
- Bobby pins
- Flexible-hold hairspray

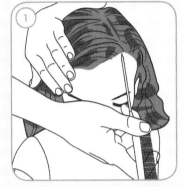

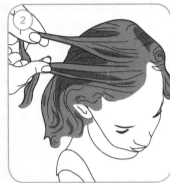

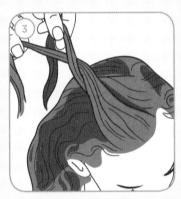

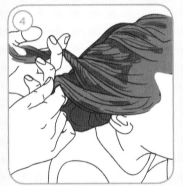

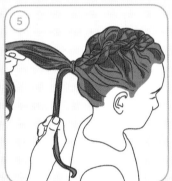

1. Brush or comb the hair. Make a side parting on the left side of the head with a rat tail comb.

2. Take a small section on the larger right side of the parting and split it in half. Hold the two sections separately in two hands.

3. Twist the hair on the right anticlockwise. Cross that section over the section on the left. Repeat, twisting the hair on the right anticlockwise and over to the left. Repeat twice more.

4. Begin to incorporate hair from underneath the twist, working towards the crown of the head. Add hair from the hairline to the right section before twisting over to the left.

5. Gather the rest of the hair and the twist into a low ponytail. Secure together with an elastic. Wrap a piece of hair from the underside of the ponytail around the elastic. Pin in place.

TOP TIP

This style works well with thicker hair, but if the hair isn't very thick, use curling tongs to add a few curls to create a bit of volume prior to creating the twisted ponytail.

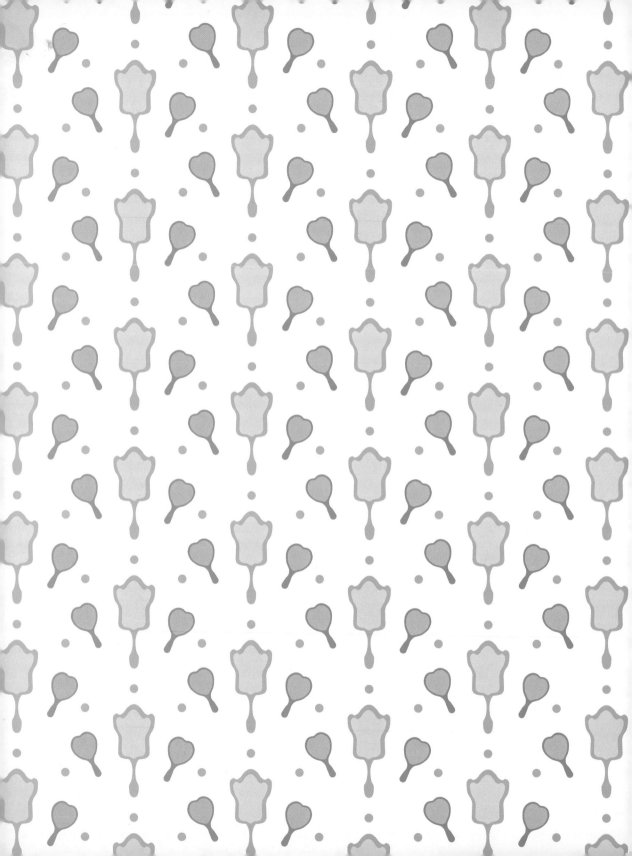

CHAPTER TWO

Braids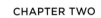

French Braid

At first glance, the classic French braid appears complicated with its intricate weave, but it is fairly simple. Once you've mastered the basics of this traditional hairstyle it will quickly become the go-to look for all of your child's casual playdates, parties or dance recitals. It's big on style and low on fuss.

DIFFICULTY LEVEL
Medium

IDEAL HAIR
Medium to long; silky texture; straight to wavy

ACCESSORIES
Dress it up with hair bows or clips.

 SEE ALSO
Heidi Braid, page 56

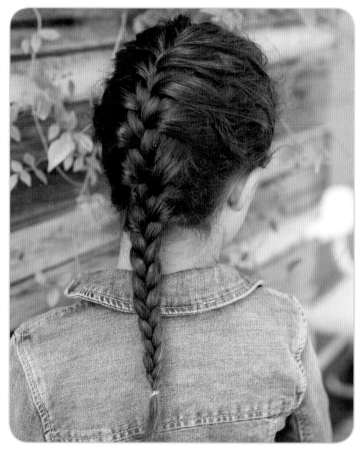

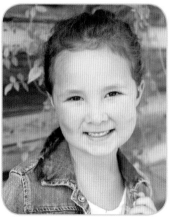

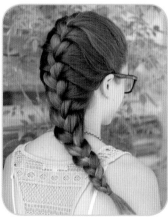

Get the look

WHAT YOU NEED

- Brush or comb
- Hair elastic

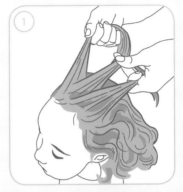
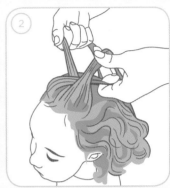
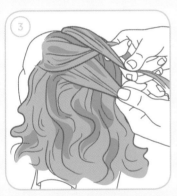
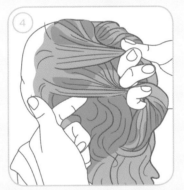
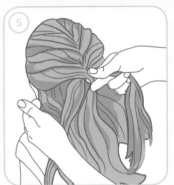

1. Brush or comb the hair. Take a small section at the hairline and divide it into three even sections.

2. Starting from the left, take that section and cross it over the centre section and under the right section, as if you are starting a basic three-strand braid.

3. Cross the right section over the centre section, holding it between the centre and left section of hair.

4. Again from the section on the left, add a small section of hair from the hairline and cross it to the centre. Repeat on the right, adding hair and crossing it to the centre.

5. Repeat these steps until there is no more hair to include on either side. Continue with a three-strand braid (see page 25) to the ends of the hair. Secure the ends with an elastic.

TOP TIP

If the hair has layers or is prone to flyaways, gently mist the hair with a spray bottle before braiding. This will help the hair go in the right direction and tame flyaways.

Side Fishtail Braid

If you have mastered the more common braids, it is time you tried the side fishtail braid. Many people are intimidated by the look of a fishtail, often fearing that it is too difficult, but once you know the technique it is quite easy. Also known as a herringbone braid, the fishtail braid works best on long thick hair with minimal layers. The best thing about a fishtail braid is that once you have set it in place, it doesn't come undone easily and it won't get frizzy.

DIFFICULTY LEVEL
Medium to hard

IDEAL HAIR
Medium to long; thick; minimal layers

ACCESSORIES
Take this style to the next level by adding a headband or some flowers across the top of the head.

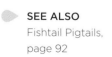
SEE ALSO
Fishtail Pigtails, page 92

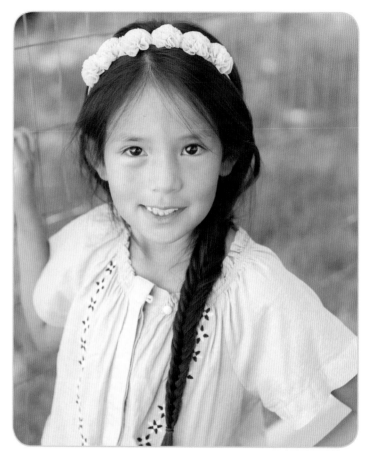

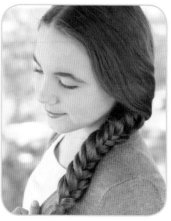

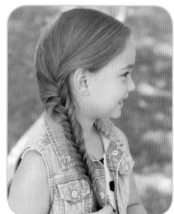

Get the look

WHAT YOU NEED

- Brush or comb
- Hair elastics
- Scissors

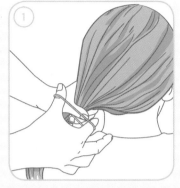
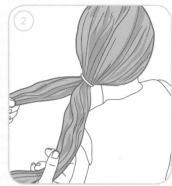
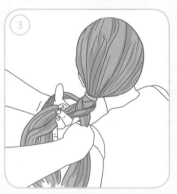
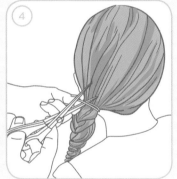
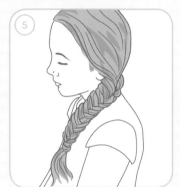

1. Brush or comb the hair until it is smooth and free from tangles. Gather the hair to the desired side into a loose ponytail. Secure into place with an elastic.

2. Divide the hair in the side ponytail in half.

3. Starting on the right side, take a small piece of hair from the outside of the section up and over to the left side. Next, on the left side, take a small piece of hair from the outside of the section up and over to the right side. Repeat these steps until you get to the ends of the hair.

4. Secure the braid at the end with an elastic. Carefully cut out the top elastic at the base of the ponytail.

5. Your braid is complete. To create a fuller fishtail braid, pinch and pull out each section of hair until you create your desired look.

TOP TIP

If the hair is silky, apply a medium-hold hairspray for extra grip while braiding to keep hair in place.

Infinity Braid

Also known as the figure eight braid, this elegant half-up, half-down look is one of the most popular braid styles because it has a unique look and it is effortless to create. This is a glam hairstyle for any formal occasion; kick it up a notch by tying a ribbon or fixing a pretty bow to the back.

DIFFICULTY LEVEL
Easy

IDEAL HAIR
Long; silky texture; straight

ACCESSORIES
Try some sparkly hair clips woven through the braid, or add a chunky headband.

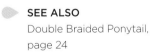 **SEE ALSO**
Double Braided Ponytail, page 24

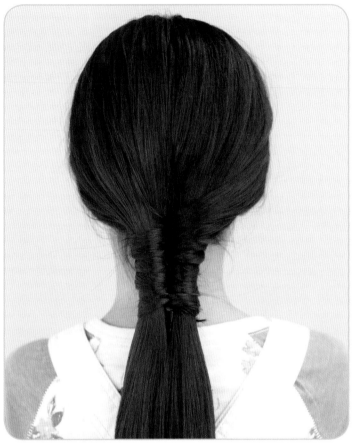

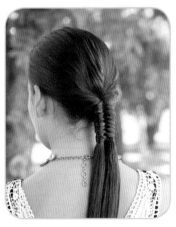

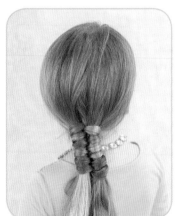

Get the look

WHAT YOU NEED

- Brush or comb
- Hair elastic

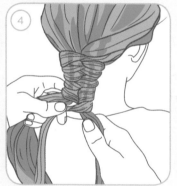
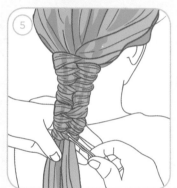
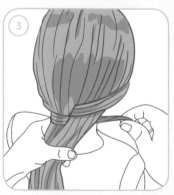
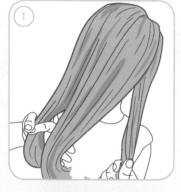
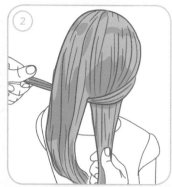

1. Brush or comb the hair. Brush the hair to the nape of the neck and divide it in half. Take a small section of hair on the right, 2.5 to 5 cm (1 to 2 inches) thick.

2. Holding the larger part to the back, take the small section of hair and cross it over the right section, underneath the left section.

3. Take the same strand of hair and wrap it over the left section, taking it over to the right, underneath the right section. You are forming a figure eight, or an infinity sign, with the hair.

4. Continue to weave the hair over and under each section, working right to left. If you run out of hair, take a small piece from inside the current section of hair to join the first section.

5. Braid until you reach your desired length. Attach a bobby pin to the ends of the hair. Push it upwards into the braid to secure it in place.

TOP TIP

If the braid does not want to hold the shape, apply a tiny bit of pomade to the hair. It will give the hair some texture, allowing it to be more easily shaped.

Braided Half-up

This cute and casual style is a favourite of busy mums. It's simple to create, looks great on all hair types and offers a stylish alternative to the everyday braid. It's also a great school day style because it neatly pulls the hair away from the face with a fun fashionable look at the back.

DIFFICULTY LEVEL
Easy

IDEAL HAIR
Medium to long; medium to thick texture; straight to wavy

ACCESSORIES
To sweeten the look, add a bow or coloured ribbon to the end of the braid. You could even apply some hair clips to the front hairline, or a headband to keep any flyaways at bay.

 SEE ALSO
Braided Bun,
page 120

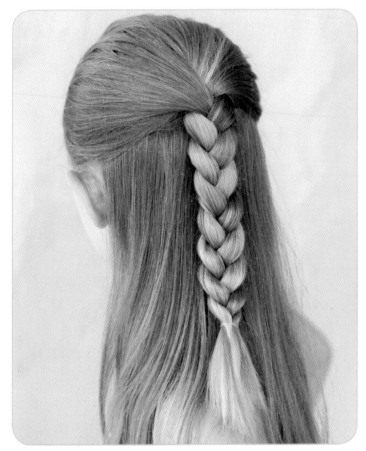

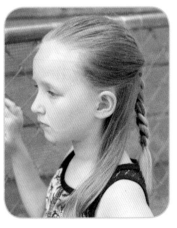

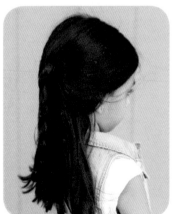

Get the look

. . . .

WHAT YOU NEED

• Brush or comb

• Hair elastic

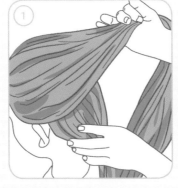
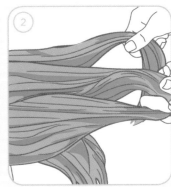
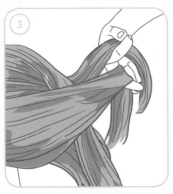
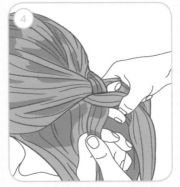
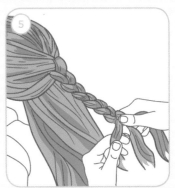

1. Brush or comb the hair until it is smooth and free from tangles. Gently brush the hair towards the back of the head. Divide the hair above the ears, separating the top from the bottom.

2. Working with the hair at the top of the head, starting from the crown, divide the hair into three sections.

3. Take the left section and cross it up and over to the middle.

4. Take the right section and cross it up and over to the middle. Repeat, working left then right, until you get to the ends.

5. Secure the end of the braid with an elastic.

TOP TIP

If the hair is silky, secure it with an elastic in a half ponytail before beginning the braid. Cut out the elastic when done styling.

Half-up Bubble Fishtail

This unique variation on the Braided Half-up is business as usual at the front, but the unexpected bubble fishtail creates a hair party at the back. This is ideal for hair of mid to long length as you need enough hair to create the bubble fishtail, and it generally requires straight to wavy hair texture too.

DIFFICULTY LEVEL
Medium

IDEAL HAIR
Medium to long; straight to wavy texture

ACCESSORIES
Finish off the fishtail with a pretty bow or bobble hair tie.

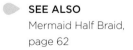 **SEE ALSO**
Mermaid Half Braid, page 62

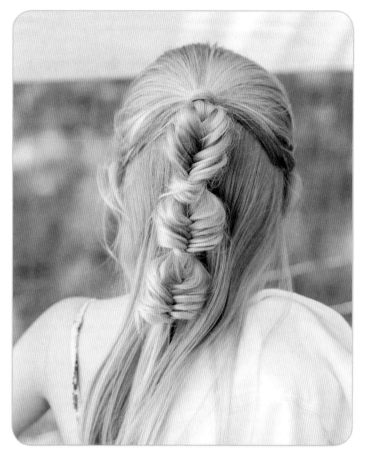

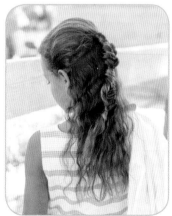

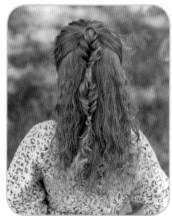

Get the look

WHAT YOU NEED

- Brush or comb
- Hair elastics
- Bobby pins

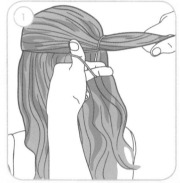
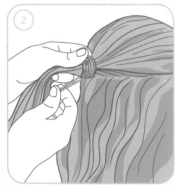
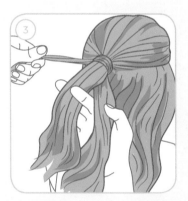
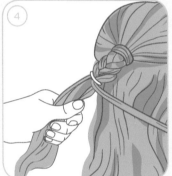
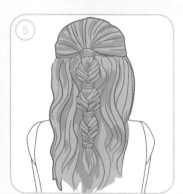

1. Brush or comb the hair. Gather the hair from the top of the head into a half-up ponytail at the crown. Secure with an elastic.

2. Wrap a small section of hair from the underside of the ponytail around the elastic. Secure the hair in place with a bobby pin.

3. Split the hair inside the ponytail in half. Take a small piece of hair from the left and cross over to the right. Then, take a small piece of hair from the right up and over to the left. Continue this movement six to eight times. Secure the ends with an elastic.

4. Cover the elastic with a small section of hair. Secure in place with a bobby pin, weaving it into the end of the braid and pushing it up into the ponytail.

5. Repeat steps 3 and 4, to create another two fishtail braids, leaving 2.5 to 5 cm (1 to 2 inches) of hair out at the end. Create the 'bubble' effect by loosening the fishtail braids slightly.

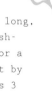

TOP TIP

If the hair is long, create many fish-tail bubbles for a dramatic effect by repeating steps 3 and 4. Leave 2.5 to 5 cm (1 to 2 inches) of hair out at the end.

Braided Headband

You will love this simple style for its fun look but also for its versatility. This is fantastic for keeping hair off the face – great for school sports days – and it's the perfect disguise if your child is growing out their fringe or needs to hide unwashed hair. This is a simple style to achieve but it gives off the illusion of effort.

DIFFICULTY LEVEL
Easy

IDEAL HAIR
Medium to long; medium to thick texture; straight to curly

ACCESSORIES
Tie a ribbon or add a pretty clip to the end of the braid.

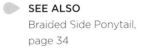

SEE ALSO
Braided Side Ponytail, page 34

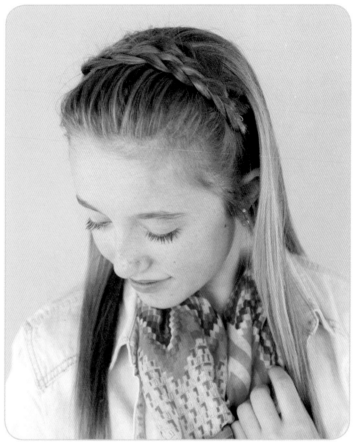

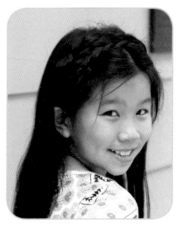

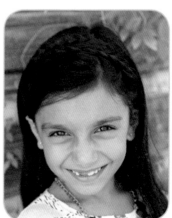

Get the look

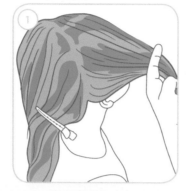
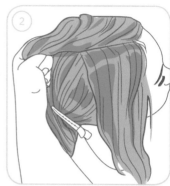
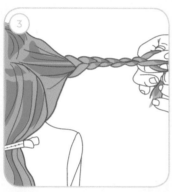
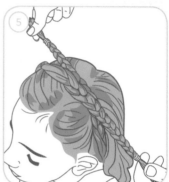
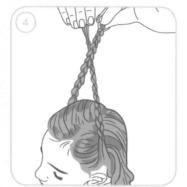

WHAT YOU NEED

- Brush or comb
- Hair clips
- Hair elastics
- Bobby pins

1. Brush or comb the hair until it is smooth and free from tangles. Split the hair from ear to ear over the top of the head and clip away the hair at the bottom.

2. Starting on the right side, create a square section from 5 to 7.5 cm (2 to 3 inches) above the ear.

3. Inside your section, split the hair off in three equal sections and begin a simple three-strand braid. Braid to the ends and secure with an elastic. Repeat steps 2 and 3 on the left side of the hair.

4. Take the ends of your braids and cross them over each other in a V-shape.

5. Place the braids down along the hairline, about 5 cm (2 inches) from the face. Secure in place with bobby pins.

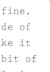

TOP TIP

If the hair is fine, stretch each side of the braid to make it fuller. A tiny bit of dry shampoo will also thicken the hair.

Heidi Braid

Also known as a milkmaid braid, the Heidi braid is a popular, glam updo. The modern Heidi braid is soft and sits towards the front of the hairline, framing the face. Despite how complicated it looks, this cute summer hairstyle is simple to create. This beautiful braid can be worn anytime but is more suited to a special occasion, dinner party or dance.

DIFFICULTY LEVEL
Medium

IDEAL HAIR
Long; medium to thick texture; straight to wavy

ACCESSORIES
Entwine a hair ribbon into the braid for a fun splash of colour.

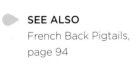

SEE ALSO
French Back Pigtails, page 94

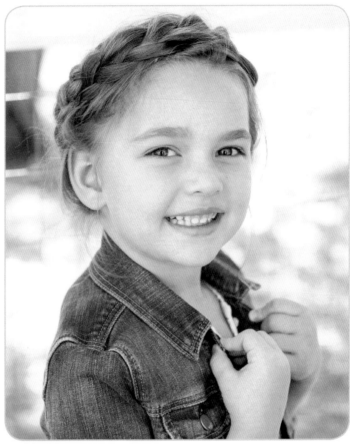

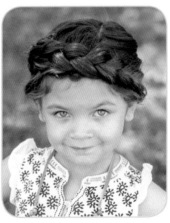

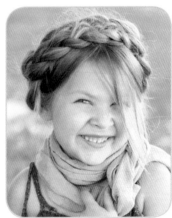

Get the look

WHAT YOU NEED

- Brush or comb
- Hair clip
- Hair elastics
- Bobby pins

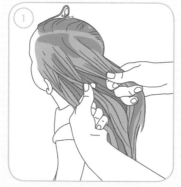

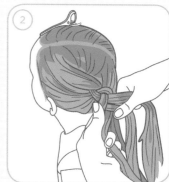

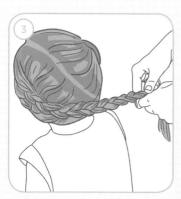

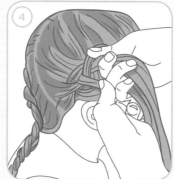

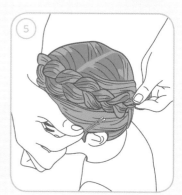

1. Brush or comb the hair. Separate into two sections diagonally from the hairline to the nape of the neck. Clip away the right section. Take some hair behind the ear of the left section and divide it into three.

2. Create an inside-out braid. Take the right section under into the middle. Take the left section under into the middle. Add hair into the braid on both sides. Repeat, directing the hair to the right around the back of the hairline until you reach the clip.

3. Continue to braid, using the three-strand braid technique (see page 25) until you reach the ends. Secure with an elastic.

4. Repeat steps 2 and 3 on the right section this time, directing the hair around towards the face.

5. Wrap the braids around the head. Pin in place with bobby pins.

TOP TIP

If the hair has short layers and sticks out of braids, create texture by adding waves. The curl will bend the hair so that it will blend back in easily.

Pull-through Braid

If you're a braiding beginner, this pull-through version is the best place to start. The name of this faux braid style comes from the many hair elastics that you 'pull' the hair through to create the look. It's a quick updo for busy school mornings but the end result is salon-worthy.

DIFFICULTY LEVEL
Easy

IDEAL HAIR
Long; minimal layers; straight to wavy

ACCESSORIES
There is a variety of options for this style, from hair clips to a big bow on the top of the pony, or a sweet headband.

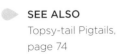
SEE ALSO
Topsy-tail Pigtails,
page 74

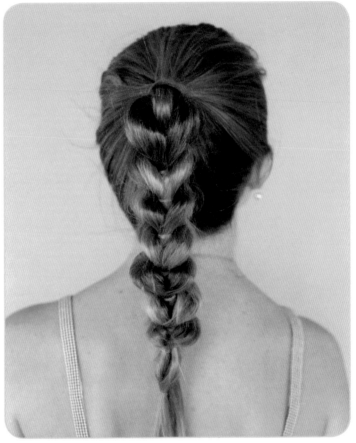

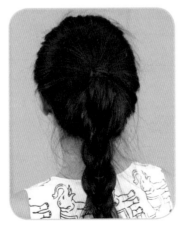

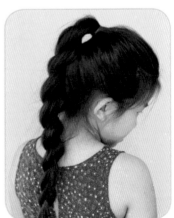

Get the look

WHAT YOU NEED

- Brush or comb
- Hair clip
- Hair elastics

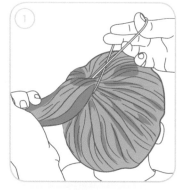
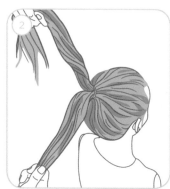
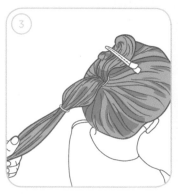
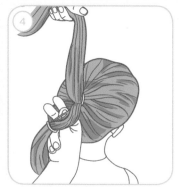
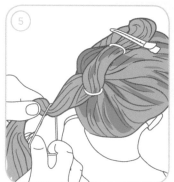

1. Brush or comb the hair until it is smooth and free from tangles. Gather the hair into a ponytail at the crown of the head. Secure in place with an elastic.

2. Divide the hair in half horizontally into two equal sections. Clip the top section away for later.

3. Add another elastic about 5 cm (2 inches) from the elastic securing the ponytail.

4. Make an opening in the middle of the two elastics. Unclip the top section and carefully pull the hair through the opening between the elastics in the bottom section.

5. Repeat steps 2 to 4 until you reach about 5 or 7.5 cm (2 or 3 inches) from the ends and secure with an elastic to finish.

TOP TIP

If the hair is slippery, add texture to it by spraying dry shampoo on the hair after forming the ponytail but before starting the braid.

Upward Lace Braid

At first glance, it looks similar to the popular waterfall braid, but this hot hairstyle is faster and easy to do too. Once you learn the simple steps, we know you'll add this to your go-to updo list for school, recitals and playdates. This braid also works well for formal events – add a beautiful big bow to the back. For the best look, style it in the middle or slightly off-centre.

DIFFICULTY LEVEL
Medium

IDEAL HAIR
Long; straight to wavy; minimal layers

ACCESSORIES
Tie a pretty ribbon over the elastic for a cute alternative.

 SEE ALSO
Heart Braid, page 68

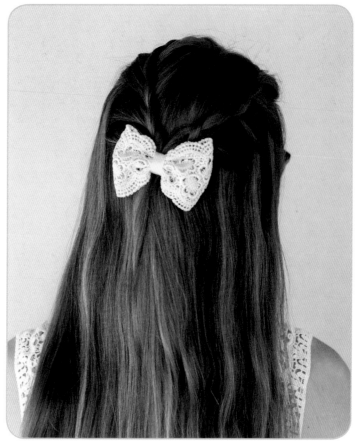

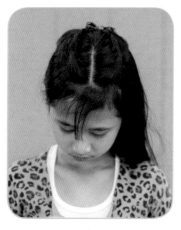

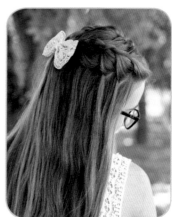

Get the look

WHAT YOU NEED
- Brush or comb
- Hair elastics
- Bobby pin

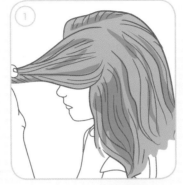
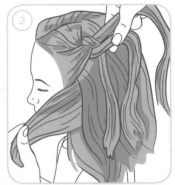
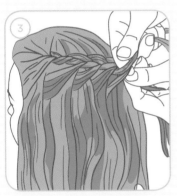
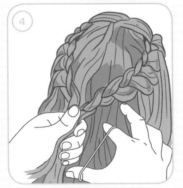
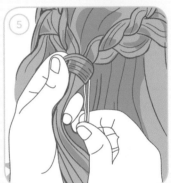

1. Brush or comb the hair. Make a parting at the middle or slightly to the side. Take a small section of hair from the hairline on the left.

2. Divide the section into three and take the left section under to the middle. Take the right section under into the middle. Add hair to the left side of the braid and take it under into the middle.

3. Take the right section under into the middle, without adding hair. Repeat, only adding hair into the left side, until you reach the middle crown of the head. Secure in place with an elastic.

4. Repeat steps 1 to 3 on the right side, but this time, add hair on the right side only. Work towards the back of the head and secure the braids together with an elastic.

5. To finish, wrap a small piece of hair around the elastic and secure in place with a bobby pin.

TOP TIP

Make sure the hair is one hundred per cent tangle free before you begin this style. If the hair is prone to tangles, add a smoothing serum while braiding. This will also tame flyaways.

Mermaid Half Braid

Also known as the floating fishtail braid, the mermaid half braid is easy and takes a few minutes! This style is ideal for straight to wavy hair, on middle to long lengths with minimal layers. It's perfect for the beach.

DIFFICULTY LEVEL
Medium

IDEAL HAIR
Medium to long; straight to barely wavy texture; minimal layers

ACCESSORIES
Add a pretty bow tie at the bottom to sweeten the deal.

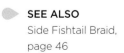 **SEE ALSO**
Side Fishtail Braid, page 46

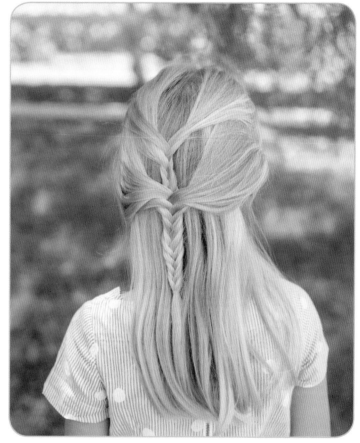

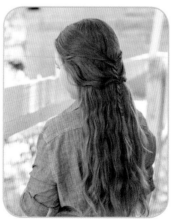

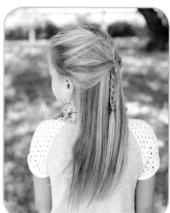

Get the look

WHAT YOU NEED

- Brush or comb
- Hair elastic

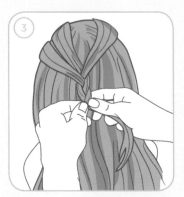
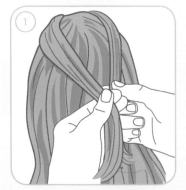
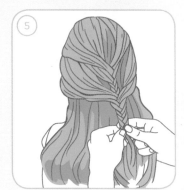
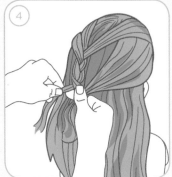
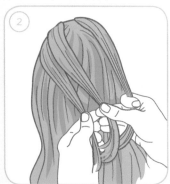

1. Brush or comb the hair. Part the hair in the middle and take a small piece of hair from each side of the parting near the hairline.

2. Separate out a piece of hair from the section on the left.

3. Using a 'floating' fishtail braiding technique, take the separated piece of hair from the left and cross it over to the right. Take a small piece of hair from the right and cross it over to the left. Work only with the sections you are holding in your hands – don't add hair from underneath.

4. Add more hair from the front of the hairline into each section, crossing the hair over left to right and then right to left.

5. Continue crossing the hair over four to six times and secure the ends with an elastic.

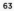

TOP TIP

This is a great style for extremely long hair for a fantastic dramatic final look.

Top Braided Bunches

Can't you see how adorable your little girl will look in this playful hairdo? You will love how practical and pretty these braided bunches are too. Your busy little lady won't have to sit still too long because the style is so easy to create. This delightful duo will survive even the most rigorous playtime without breaking a sweat.

DIFFICULTY LEVEL
Easy

IDEAL HAIR
Long; afro texture to medium coarseness; thick

ACCESSORIES
Brighten up this hairstyle with a pop of colour via bows or a headband.

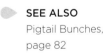 **SEE ALSO**
Pigtail Bunches, page 82

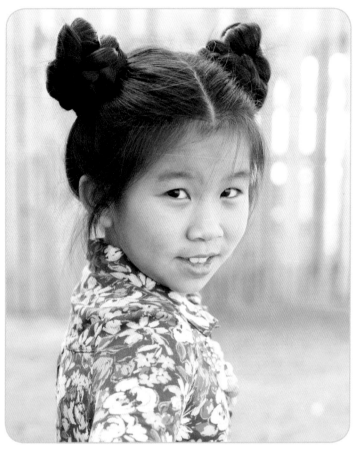

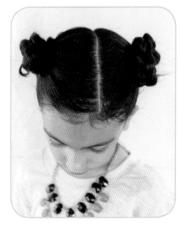

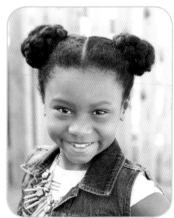

Get the look

WHAT YOU NEED

- Brush or comb
- Hair elastics
- Bobby pins

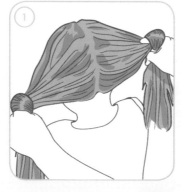
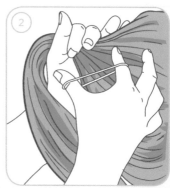
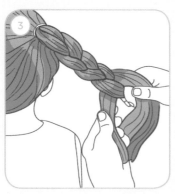
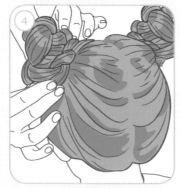
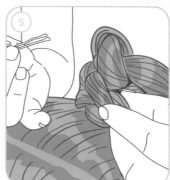

1. Brush or comb the hair until it is smooth and free from tangles. Divide the hair in half into two equal sections.

2. Gather the hair into a ponytail on each side at the high crown. Secure in place with elastics.

3. Divide the hair in each ponytail into three equal sections. Braid using the three-strand braid technique (see page 25), working right to left. Secure the ends of each braided ponytail with an elastic.

4. Take each braid and wrap it around the elastic at the crown, forming a bunch on each side.

5. Secure each bunch in place with bobby pins as you wrap.

TOP TIP

If the braids are small, feel free to stretch out the braid prior to creating your bun so it will have a fuller look.

Elsa Braid

Children across the world have been gripped by the *Frozen* phenomenon, and they can't seem to 'Let It Go', no matter how much Elsa sings. But crooning along to the movie isn't enough for our little princesses; they want their locks to look the part too. Now the iconic Elsa braid is a global sensation. To make this authentic, you need to recreate the slightly teased 'pouf' at the front. This height is the difference between a regular braid and a Queen Elsa one. This style of braid requires long, thick hair, but of course mothers of a *Frozen*-obsessed daughter can make it work on their daughter's hair.

DIFFICULTY LEVEL
Medium

IDEAL HAIR
Long; thick texture; wavy

ACCESSORIES
Spray with a little glitter to add a faux icy look to the hair.

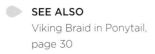 **SEE ALSO**
Viking Braid in Ponytail, page 30

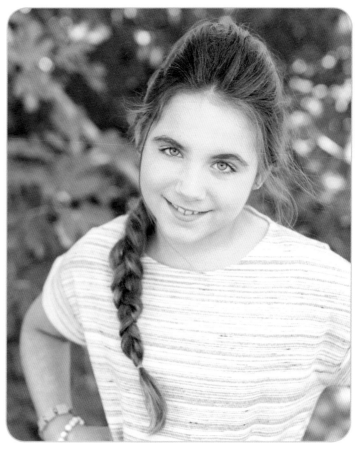

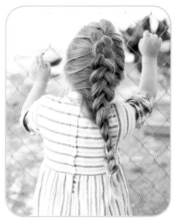

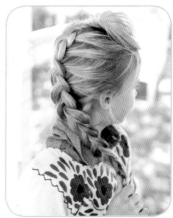

Get the look

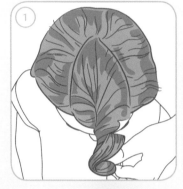
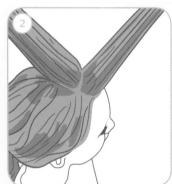
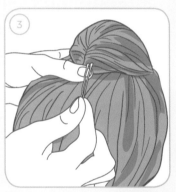
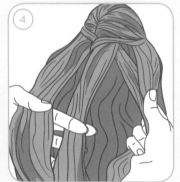
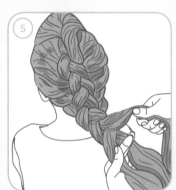

WHAT YOU NEED

- Brush or comb
- Hair clip
- Bobby pin
- Hair elastic

1. Brush or comb the hair. Take a small triangle section of hair from the crown to the forehead. Clip the rest of the hair away.

2. To create the 'pouf', take horizontal sections inside the triangle, and tease with your comb at the root area.

3. Take the teased hair and pull it back and secure in place with a bobby pin by twisting and pushing the triangle section forward.

4. Unclip the rest of the hair. Divide it into three sections. Begin an inside-out braid (see page 57), working right then left, taking the hair under and into the middle. Add hair on both sides, braiding close to the scalp.

5. Braid the rest of the hair, braiding under, rather than over, using the three-strand braid technique (see page 25), until you reach the ends. Secure in place with an elastic.

TOP TIP

If the hair is fine, you can use a salt spray for added volume. This will give fullness at the roots so you can get a true Elsa braid.

Heart Braid

This gorgeous hairdo is the ultimate symbol of love. A fun twist on the traditional braid, it's for those who love the look and versatility of half-up, half-down styles. It's simple to create and keeps your child's hair neatly off the face while still looking pretty.

DIFFICULTY LEVEL
Medium

IDEAL HAIR
Medium to long; fine to thick; straight to wavy

ACCESSORIES
Swap your everyday elastic with a fun one. We love flowery hair ties – they add even more romance to this style.

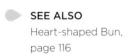 **SEE ALSO**
Heart-shaped Bun, page 116

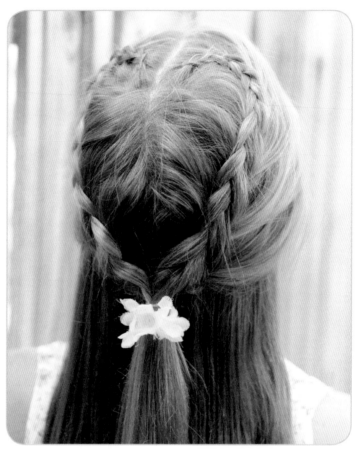

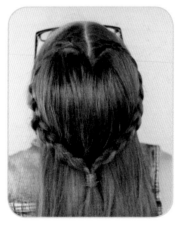

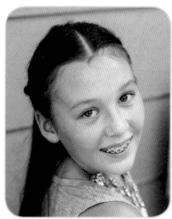

Get the look

WHAT YOU NEED

- Brush or comb
- Hair clip
- Hair elastics

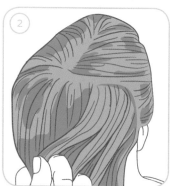
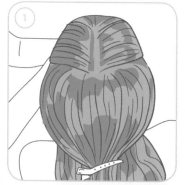
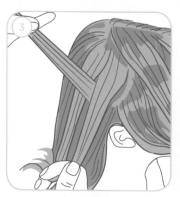
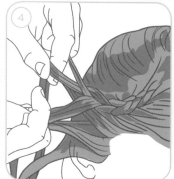
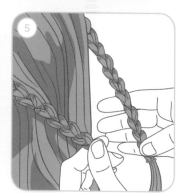

1. Brush or comb the hair. Make a centre parting, and then create a half-heart shape at the crown on both sides of the parting, ensuring each side of the heart is even. Clip the hair inside the heart away.

2. Starting on one side at the top centre of your heart-shaped section, take a 2.5-cm (1-inch) section and divide it in three.

3. Using the inside-out braid technique (see page 57), take the right section of hair up and under into the middle. Then take the left section up and under into the middle.

4. Add hair to the section closest to the hairline only as you braid. Continue to braid until you get to the bottom tip of your heart. Secure the ends with an elastic.

5. Repeat on the other side. When you reach the tip of the heart, connect the braids, securing with an elastic, and release the clip.

TOP TIP

If the hair is slippery with lots of flyaways, use a light mist product before you begin to braid. This will allow for a good grip on the tiny sections of hair.

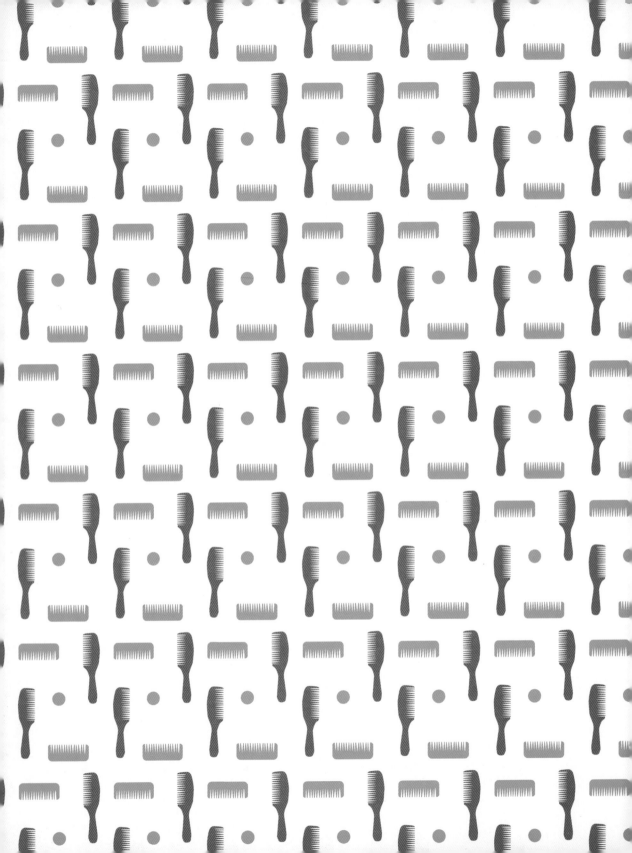

CHAPTER THREE

Pigtails

Messy Low Pigtails

These messy pigtails are very easy to tie and are one of our favourites for those mornings when you need a look that's simple, yet pulled together at the same time. The slightly messy shape of these pigtails is the best part because it requires little to no styling. Let your child's hair be wild and free. This style is great for wavy to curly hair as you already have the ideal texture to create a tousled effect. For this style your child should have mid- to long-length hair with a fine to medium thickness. You could try it out on shorter hair – you will have shorter pigtails.

DIFFICULTY LEVEL
Easy

IDEAL HAIR
Medium to long; fine to medium texture; wavy or curly

ACCESSORIES
Some coloured clips would be cute on either side of the hairline. Clips are also great for keeping shorter fringes or pesky flyaways out of your child's eyes.

SEE ALSO
Messy Low Ponytail, page 26

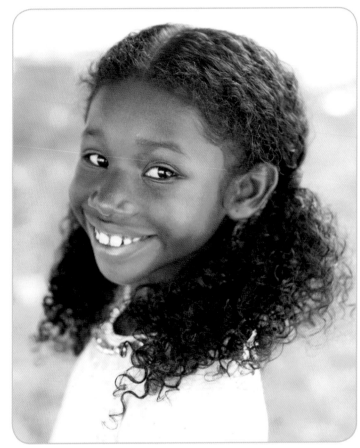

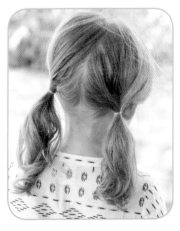

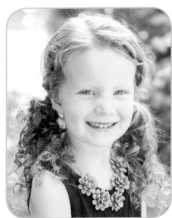

Get the look

WHAT YOU NEED

- Brush or comb
- Hair elastics
- Bobby pins

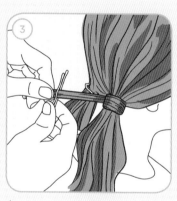
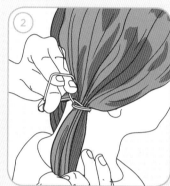
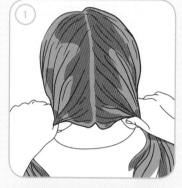
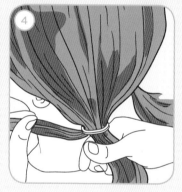
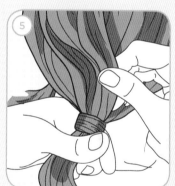

1. Brush or comb the hair until it is smooth and free from tangles. Make a centre parting.

2. Starting on the right side, gather the hair into a low ponytail. Secure in place with an elastic behind the ear. Repeat on the left side.

3. Cover the right hair elastic by taking a small section of hair from the underside of the ponytail and wrapping around the elastic. Secure the hair in place with a bobby pin.

4. Repeat step 3 on the left ponytail.

5. Hold the base of each ponytail, and pinch and pull hair in an upwards direction to create a messy texture.

TOP TIP

If the hair is straight and you want a messier style, curl the hair prior to creating the pigtails. This will help give the hair a curly texture for that messy look.

Topsy-tail Pigtails

This modern twist on the quintessential preschool pigtail makes it a school day staple for most mums. It works well on all hair types, and your little girl can run around the school playground and those pigtails will stay in place all day.

DIFFICULTY LEVEL
Easy

IDEAL HAIR
Medium to long; fine to thick; straight and wavy

ACCESSORIES
You can use a dainty headband to up the cute factor, and hair bows or hair clips always look cute for this style.

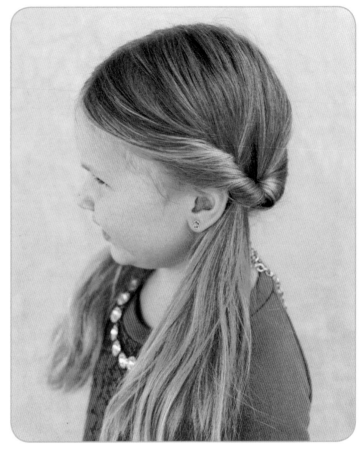

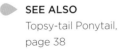
SEE ALSO
Topsy-tail Ponytail,
page 38

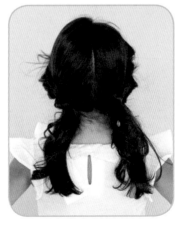

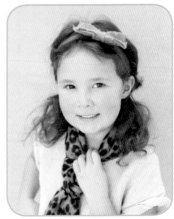

Get the look

WHAT YOU NEED
- Brush or comb
- Hair elastics
- Bobby pins

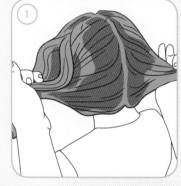
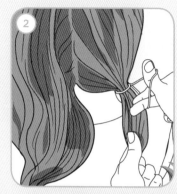
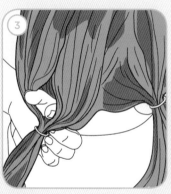
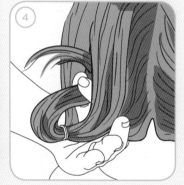
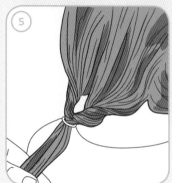

1. Brush or comb the hair until it is smooth and free from tangles. Make a centre parting.

2. Gather all the hair on one side of the parting directly behind the ear into a low ponytail. Secure in place with an elastic. Repeat on the other side.

3. Loosen each ponytail to allow the hair to be pulled through. Split the low loose ponytail in half behind the elastic, making a hole with your fingers.

4. Thread the end of the ponytail through the loop.

5. Pull gently on the end of the ponytail to secure into place. To finish, wrap a piece of hair from the ponytail around the elastic and secure in place with a bobby pin. Repeat on the other side.

TOP TIP

If you have a topsy-tail tool (see page 38), you can use this to turn the pigtails upside down, instead of using your fingers.

Half-up Pigtails

The grateful grin from your happy child in pigtails will be more than worth the minimal effort required to create them. Half-up pigtails are easy for the mum or dad with little to no hair experience – all you need are hair elastics, a clip and a comb. Take your child to the cinema, a birthday party or to their favourite theme park in this cute kiddie favourite. It's pretty but tough so it can withstand hours of playtime without the need for touch-ups or a redo.

DIFFICULTY LEVEL
Easy

IDEAL HAIR
Short to medium; fine to medium texture; straight

ACCESSORIES
Style the look with bows or ribbons tied to each pigtail.

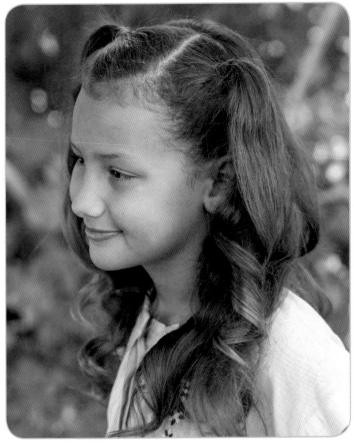

 SEE ALSO
Half Ponytail,
page 18

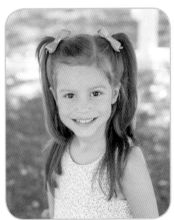

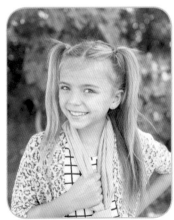

Get the look

WHAT YOU NEED

- Brush or comb
- Hair clip
- Hair elastics

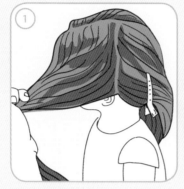

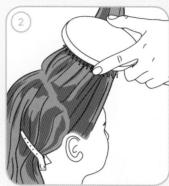

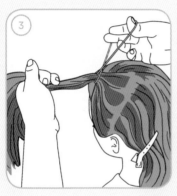

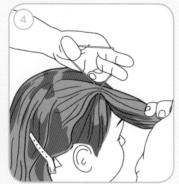

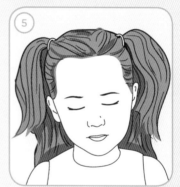

1. Brush or comb the hair until it is smooth and free from tangles. Make a centre parting. Divide the hair from ear to ear, creating two sections in front of the ears. Clip the back hair away.

2. Brush the hair up above the ear by 5 to 7.5 cm (2 to 3 inches).

3. Gather into a ponytail, tightly securing the hair in place with an elastic.

4. Repeat on the opposite side.

5. Remove the clip from the back hair and brush through.

TOP TIP

Create a more formal half-up pigtail look by curling the hair before creating the pigtails. Curl the hair in small sections with 2.5-cm (1-inch) curling tongs.

High Pigtails

Take the standard pigtail to new heights with this adorable update. It's a different look from the usual pigtail styles we know and love because of its unique positioning high up on the crown. Your little girl's hair will bounce along while she's having fun at school, with friends or at a party.

DIFFICULTY LEVEL
Easy

IDEAL HAIR
Medium to long; straight or wavy

ACCESSORIES
Add some jaunty hair ribbons or mini bows to the top of each pigtail for extra fun.

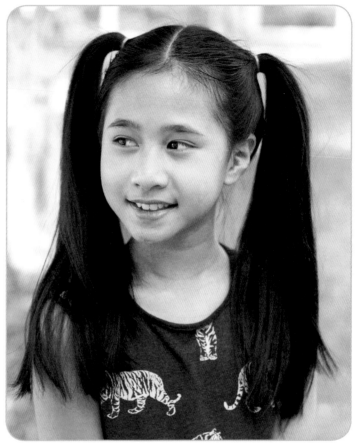

SEE ALSO
High Crown Ponytail, page 16

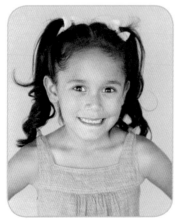

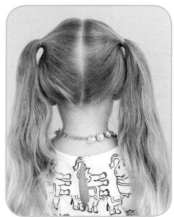

Get the look

WHAT YOU NEED

- Brush or comb
- Rat tail comb
- Hair elastics

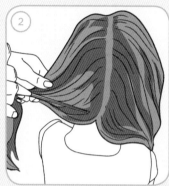

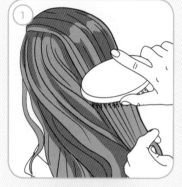

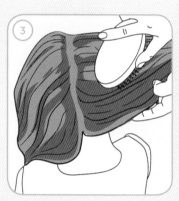

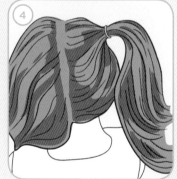

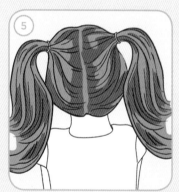

1. Brush or comb the hair until it is smooth and free from tangles.
2. Make a centre parting with a rat tail comb.
3. Starting on one side of the head, gather the hair into a high ponytail, brushing it up 5 to 7.5 cm (2 to 3 inches) above the ear.
4. Secure in place with an elastic.
5. Repeat on the other side.

TOP TIP

To achieve a fuller pigtail, create volume by curling the pigtail using 2.5-cm (1-inch) curling tongs, clamping the hair down at the middle and easing the hair through the tongs.

Zigzag Pigtails

Give the regular pigtail a fun
and funky twist with this cool
zigzag parting. It's easy for
those mums who still want the
convenience of the classic
pigtail style, but want to spice
up the style with a more
defined parting. Once you
master the zigzag form, this
pigtail version can be done in
minutes. It really is that easy,
which is why it's a great school
day look, but also a fantastic
fashion style for every
casual occasion.

DIFFICULTY LEVEL
Easy

IDEAL HAIR
Medium to long; fine to thick;
wavy to curly

ACCESSORIES
Take this look to the next level
with some hair bows, fashion
clips or ribbon.

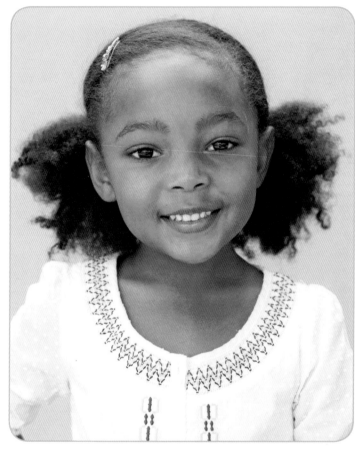

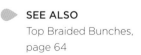 **SEE ALSO**
Top Braided Bunches,
page 64

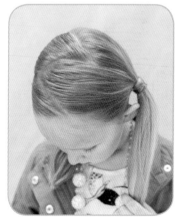 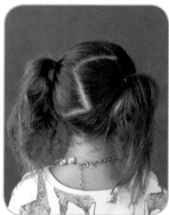

Get the look

WHAT YOU NEED

- Brush or comb
- Rat tail comb
- Hair clip
- Hair elastics

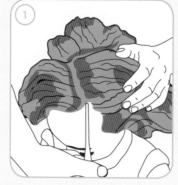

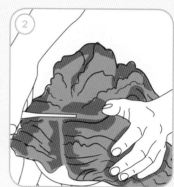

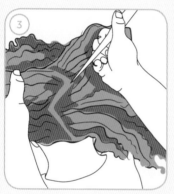

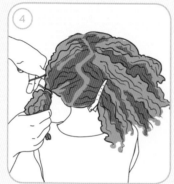

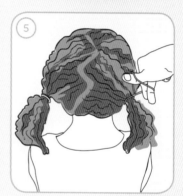

1. Brush or comb the hair until it is smooth and free from tangles. Take a rat tail comb and, beginning at the front of the hairline, start to create a 2.5- to 5-cm (1- to 2-inch) zigzag parting.

2. Slide the comb from the hairline to 5 cm (2 inches) away from the centre. Turn the zigzag parting 90 degrees, moving the rat tail comb about 5 cm (2 inches) back towards the ear.

3. Alternating taking the parting to the right and the left, continue the zigzag until you reach the nape of the neck.

4. Clip away the hair on the right and gather the hair on the left into a pigtail behind the ear. Secure with an elastic.

5. Remove the clip and gather the hair on the right into a pigtail behind the ear. Secure with an elastic.

TOP TIP

It might be easier to create a straight parting using the ends of a weaving comb due to its sharp edges.

Pigtail Bunches

This variation on the typical pigtail is a great option when you want a sophisticated style. Pigtail bunches generally work best on thick and curly hair textures because the curl gives the hair fullness. Mid- to long-length hair is preferable so you can create a large 'bunch'. If you want it to last the whole day, use a little hairspray and ensure the bobby pins are secure.

DIFFICULTY LEVEL
Easy

IDEAL HAIR
Medium to long; thick and curly texture

ACCESSORIES
Add some cute clips to each pigtail.

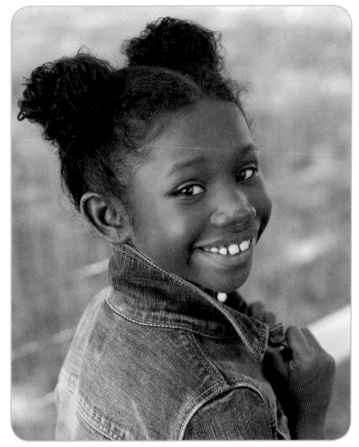

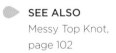 **SEE ALSO**
Messy Top Knot, page 102

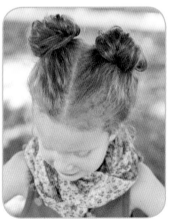

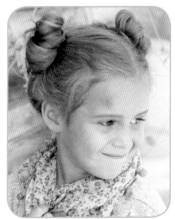

Get the look

WHAT YOU NEED

- Brush or comb
- Hair clip
- Hair elastics
- Bobby pins

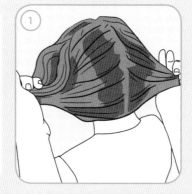

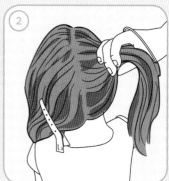

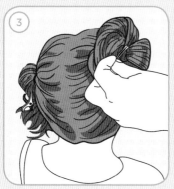

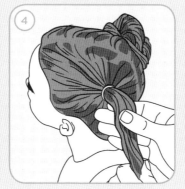

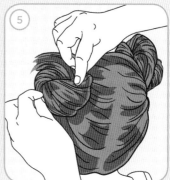

1. Brush or comb the hair until it is smooth and free from tangles. Make a centre parting. Clip one section away.

2. Pull the hair up 5 to 7.5 cm (2 to 3 inches) above the ear to create a side ponytail. Secure in place with an elastic.

3. Twist the hair, wrapping it around the elastic, to create a 'bunch'. Secure it in place with a couple of bobby pins.

4. Unclip the other section of hair and gather it into a side ponytail. Secure it in place with an elastic.

5. Repeat step 3, creating the bunch on this side.

TOP TIP

If the hair is fine, tease the hair in the pigtails to create extra fullness within the bunch.

Shirley Temple Pigtails

Shirley Temple was a dimple-faced and determined child star who sang and danced her way into our hearts. You can recreate her iconic Hollywood hairstyle on your own little star. This look is adorable and easy to do, but you might need to set aside a little more time to perfect the curls. These pigtails are perfect for young girls with fine hair that is mid- to long-length. Any shorter and you won't be able to create those curls on each side.

DIFFICULTY LEVEL
Medium

IDEAL HAIR
Medium to long; fine texture; wavy to curly

ACCESSORIES
Get that iconic Shirley Temple look by adding a ribbon tied as a headband to this style.

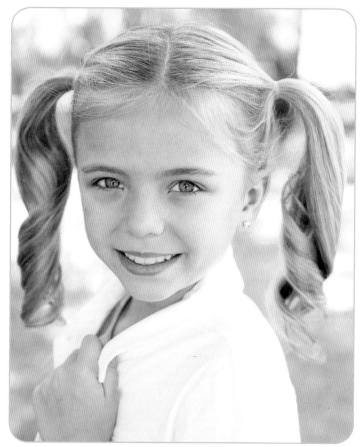

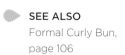 **SEE ALSO**
Formal Curly Bun, page 106

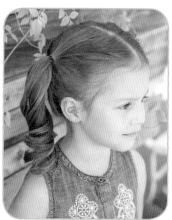

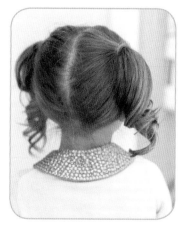

Get the look

WHAT YOU NEED

- Brush or comb
- Rat tail comb
- Hair elastics
- Medium-hold hairspray
- 2.5-cm (1-inch) curling tongs

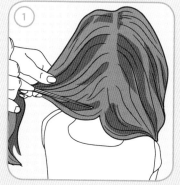
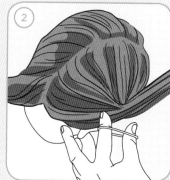
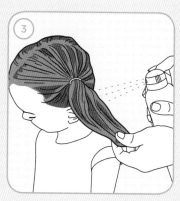
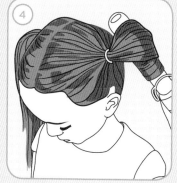
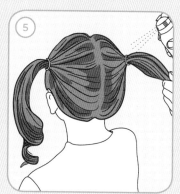

1. Brush or comb the hair until it is smooth and free from tangles. Make a centre parting with a rat tail comb.

2. Gather the hair into a ponytail on each side of the parting, 2.5 cm (1 inch) above the ear. Secure each ponytail with an elastic.

3. Spray the hair with a medium-hold hairspray.

4. Take your 2.5-cm (1-inch) curling tongs and curl the hair at the base of one ponytail, easing the hair through the hair tongs. Hold hair in curling tongs for a few seconds, and release. Add a tiny bit more medium-hold hairspray to hold the curl.

5. Repeat on the other side.

TOP TIP

If the hair is resistant to holding curls, add a light mousse and blow dry for extra hold.

Twisted Back Pigtails

This twisted style has an intricate look but it takes just minutes to pull together. The twists tame the hair away from the face to create a trendy ridge before the hair freely falls at the back. This fashionable, foolproof style looks good whatever the occasion.

DIFFICULTY LEVEL
Easy

IDEAL HAIR
Medium to long; thick texture; curly

ACCESSORIES
You can use coloured bobby pins to pretty it up, but hair bows, flower clips or a headband will look great too.

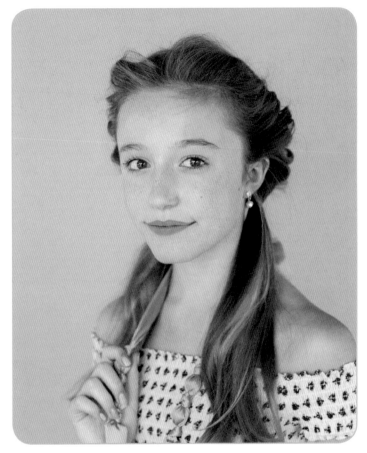

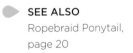
SEE ALSO
Ropebraid Ponytail, page 20

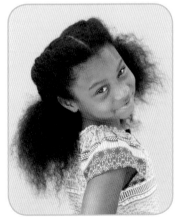

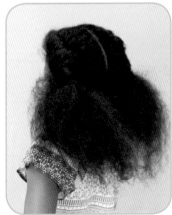

Get the look

WHAT YOU NEED

- Brush or comb
- Hair elastics

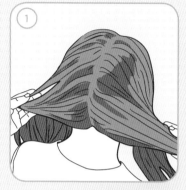

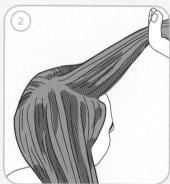

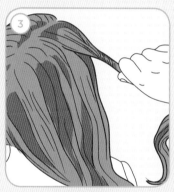

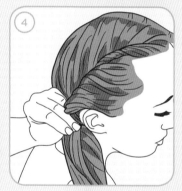

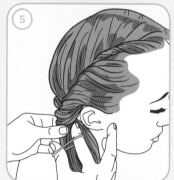

1. Brush or comb the hair until it is smooth and free from tangles. Make a centre parting.

2. Starting on one side, take a section of hair from the parting to the hairline at the front of the head.

3. Starting at the hairline on the right, twist the hair anticlockwise, moving down the section away from the face.

4. Continue your twist from the front of the hairline to the back of the ear, adding hair into the twist as you go.

5. When you reach the side nape of the neck, secure the end of the pigtail with an elastic. Repeat, twisting clockwise, on the left.

TOP TIP

If the hair is very thick, you may need to make tighter twists to ensure it stays in place.

Curly Voluminous Pigtails

Your little girl will love this edgy update on the sophisticated classic. This curly voluminous version gives pretty pigtails a little attitude with a tousled and slightly messy flurry of curls on each side. It's stylish yet speedy, so it's a good one for the morning school rush, but it's so cute you'll want to recreate it for fun playdates, birthday parties and functions.

DIFFICULTY LEVEL
Easy

IDEAL HAIR
Medium to long; thick texture; curly

ACCESSORIES
If you want to pretty up this style, add a bow or hair clip to each pigtail. You can also tie a coloured ribbon around each one.

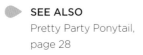 **SEE ALSO**
Pretty Party Ponytail, page 28

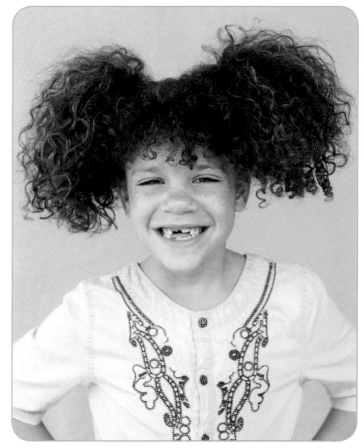

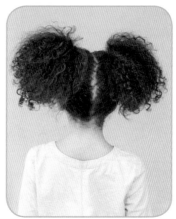 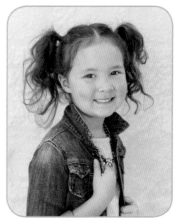

Get the look

WHAT YOU NEED

- Brush or comb
- Hair clip
- Hair elastics
- Lightweight hairspray

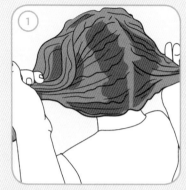
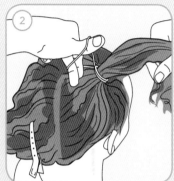
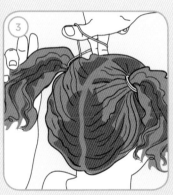
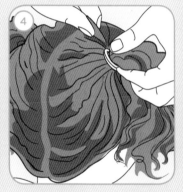
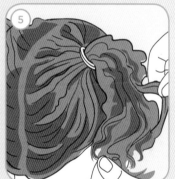

1. Brush or comb the hair until it is smooth and free from tangles. Make a centre parting. Clip away the left section for later.

2. Gather the hair on the right side into a high ponytail and then pull it into a side ponytail. Secure in place with an elastic.

3. Unclip the left section and gather the hair into a high ponytail and then pull it into a side ponytail. Secure in place with an elastic.

4. Hold the base of each ponytail, and pinch and pull hair in an upwards direction to create a messy texture.

5. Finger tease each pigtail to create volume and fullness. Spritz with lightweight hairspray to finish.

TOP TIP

If the hair isn't naturally curly, add a few curls using 2.5-cm (1-inch) curling tongs. This will add the curl and volume to create this style.

Ropebraid Pigtails

From toddlers to teens, the ropebraid is a classic. This hairdo isn't only for the playground – edgier versions have been a hit on the catwalk. It's time to bring the cord-like braids back and relive your own younger years with your little girl. Ropebraid pigtails are suited to mid- to long-length hair with thin to medium texture. They are great for swimming lessons because the hair is completely out of the way and secure.

DIFFICULTY LEVEL
Easy

IDEAL HAIR
Medium to long; thin to medium texture

ACCESSORIES
Team your ropebraid pigtails with coiled headbands for a touch of fancy, or ball hair ties.

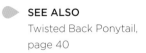

SEE ALSO
Twisted Back Ponytail, page 40

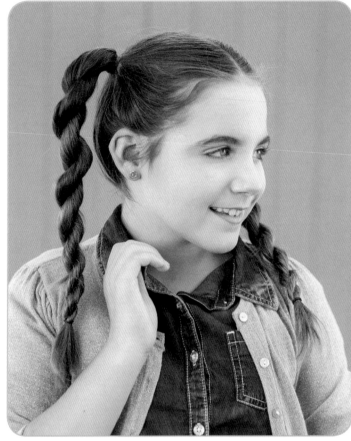

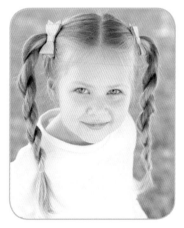

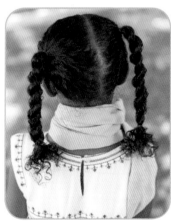

Get the look

WHAT YOU NEED

- Brush or comb
- Rat tail comb
- Hair elastics

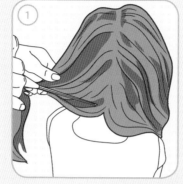

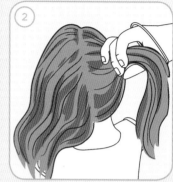

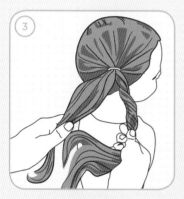

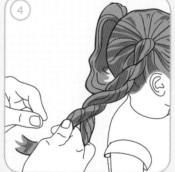

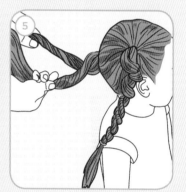

1. Brush or comb the hair until it is smooth and free from tangles. Make a centre parting with a rat tail comb.

2. Create a side ponytail between the ear and the crown. Secure with an elastic. Repeat on the other side.

3. Separate the ponytail into two sections. Twist one section clockwise.

4. Take that section up and over to the left. Twist the other section clockwise and take it up and over to the left.

5. Repeat the technique until you get to the ends of the hair. Secure with an elastic. Repeat on the other side.

TOP TIP

For sleek pigtails, lightly mist the hair with some water or leave-in conditioner before beginning the ropebraids. This will smooth any flyaways as well as create a silky texture to the braids.

Fishtail Pigtails

If you're a fan of the popular fishtail styles, you'll love this fashionable fusion. This fishtail-meets-pigtail mash-up adds some much needed interest to the standard look. Once you master the fishtail braid, the hairstyle is really simple to create. It's a fun update on the typical pigtail styles.

DIFFICULTY LEVEL
Medium

IDEAL HAIR
Long; fine to thick; straight to wavy

ACCESSORIES
Use some colourful hair bows or hair clips for added flair. A stylish headband is also a great addition.

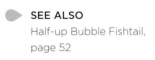 **SEE ALSO**
Half-up Bubble Fishtail, page 52

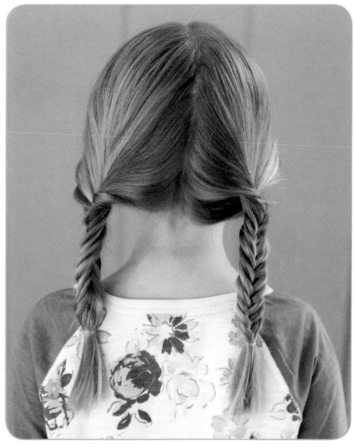

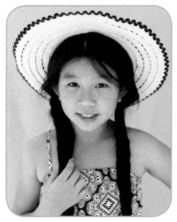

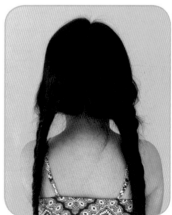

Get the look

WHAT YOU NEED

- Brush or comb
- Hair elastics
- Scissors

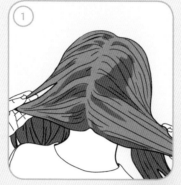
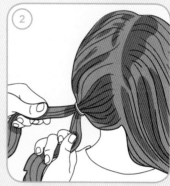
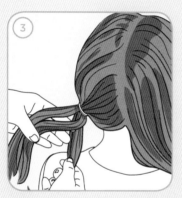
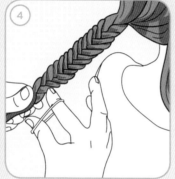
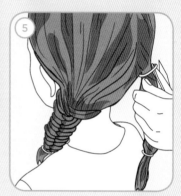

1. Brush or comb the hair until it is smooth and free from tangles. Make a centre parting.

2. Gather the hair below the ear on the left side to create a low ponytail. Secure into place with an elastic.

3. Working on the left side, divide the hair in the ponytail into two equal sections. Take a small piece of hair from the right side and cross it over to the left side. Take a small piece of hair from the left side and cross it over to the right side.

4. Continue braiding until you reach the ends. Secure the braid in place with an elastic. Repeat steps 2 to 4 on the other side.

5. Using scissors, cut out the elastic at the top of each braid.

TOP TIP

To make the hair appear fuller, pull out each individual section inside the fishtail pigtail braid.

French Back Pigtails

French braids have always been
a popular way to tie hair back,
especially during the summer.
Your child will need at least
mid- to long-length hair and it
generally suits wavy to curly
hair with medium to thick
texture. French back pigtails
are perfect for school, birthday
parties, summer fun days at the
beach or any time when there
will be high intensity activity,
because this look will stay put
all day.

DIFFICULTY LEVEL
Medium

IDEAL HAIR
Medium to long; medium to
thick texture; wavy to curly

ACCESSORIES
Attach some fun bows, ribbons
or cute summery hair clips to
the ends of these pigtails.

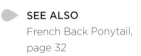 **SEE ALSO**
French Back Ponytail,
page 32

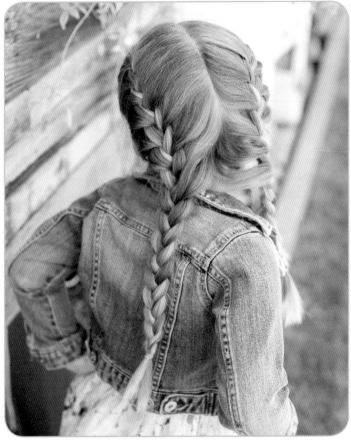

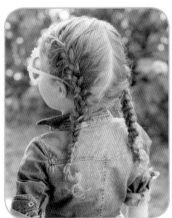

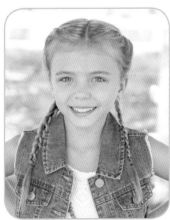

Get the look

WHAT YOU NEED

- Brush or comb
- Hair clip
- Hair elastics

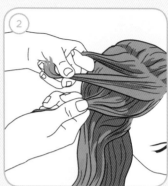

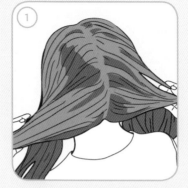

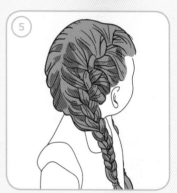

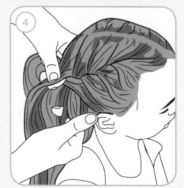

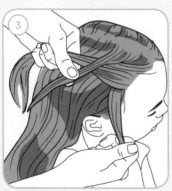

1. Brush or comb the hair. Make a centre parting.

2. Take a small section from the right side of the parting at the forehead and divide it into three even sections.

3. Starting with the right section, cross it over to the middle. Cross the left section over to the middle. The section that started in the middle is now on the right, the right section is now on the left and the left section moves to the middle.

4. Add hair from the hairline into the right section. Take it and the added hair to the middle. Repeat, adding hair to the sections on each side and moving right to left until you get to the nape of the neck. Continue with the basic three-strand braid technique (see page 25) down to the ends. Secure with an elastic.

5. Repeat steps 3 and 4 to create a French braid on the other side.

TOP TIP

If the curls are unruly and sticking out of the braids, try lightly misting the hair with a water spray bottle to help tame flyaways.

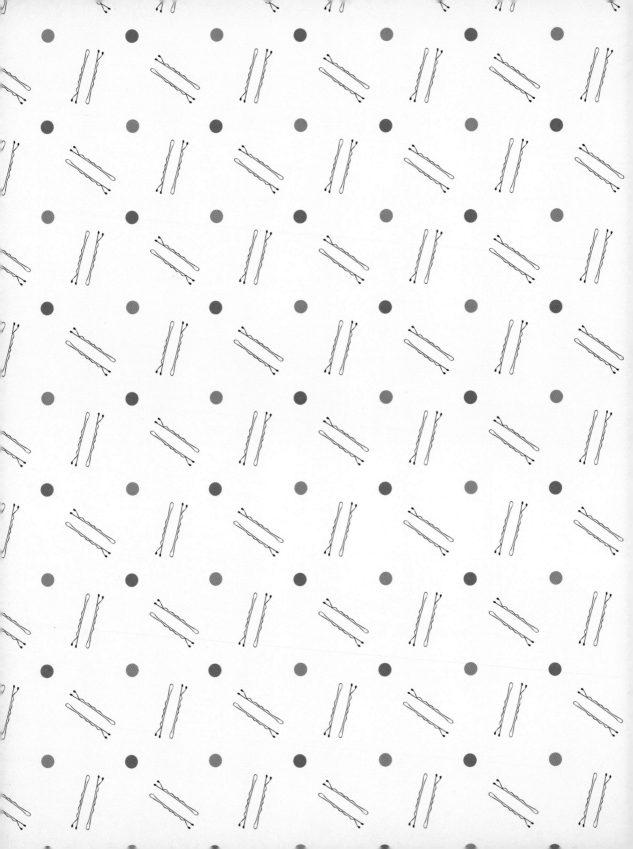

CHAPTER FOUR

Buns and Twists

Side Twists

Transform your child's hair into a bold statement with these quick and easy side twists. This is the best hair hack for the morning school runs because it's simple to create in a short amount of time. It's a great option for girls growing out their fringe because it pulls the hair away from their eyes.

DIFFICULTY LEVEL
Easy

IDEAL HAIR
Collarbone to medium; wavy or curly

ACCESSORIES
Have fun with a variety of hair clips, hair bows or even a decorated hair comb.

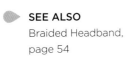
SEE ALSO
Braided Headband, page 54

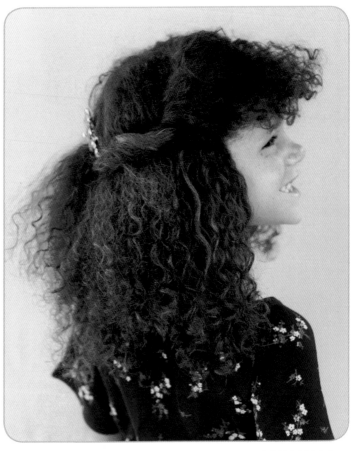

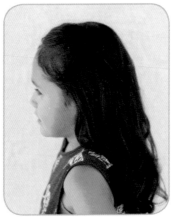

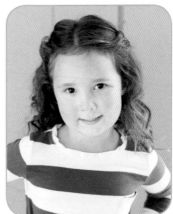

Get the look

WHAT YOU NEED

- Brush or comb
- Bobby pins

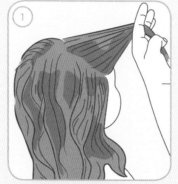

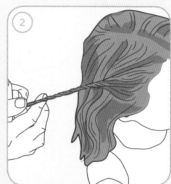

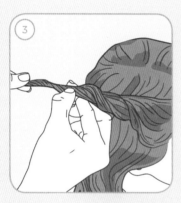

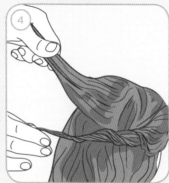

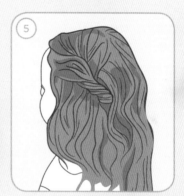

1. Brush or comb the hair until it is smooth and free from tangles. Take a small section of hair from the front of the hairline on one side, 5 cm (2 inches) from the face.

2. Twist the section anticlockwise away from the face from roots to ends until it gets to the back of the head.

3. Loosen the twist slightly, scrunching and teasing it with your fingers for some volume.

4. Direct the end of the twist to the back of the head. Pick up a piece of hair from the crown and secure your twist in place with a bobby pin directly under the piece of hair you picked up. Lay the hair back down over the end of the twist.

5. Repeat steps 1 to 4, to create the side twist on the other side.

TOP TIP

If the hair is thin and doesn't have a lot of body, curl it prior to adding your twists for additional volume and texture.

Twisty Bun

Have you run out of styling options for your buns? This twist is big on style and low on fuss. It's chic and it doesn't take much time to pull off. The twisty bun is great for thick curly hair because you already have fullness from the curls. You will need longer length hair to create this look but it should also work on shorter hair – the bun won't be as big.

DIFFICULTY LEVEL
Easy

IDEAL HAIR
Medium to long; thick texture; wavy to curly

ACCESSORIES
Tie a big bow around this bun for a really fun look.

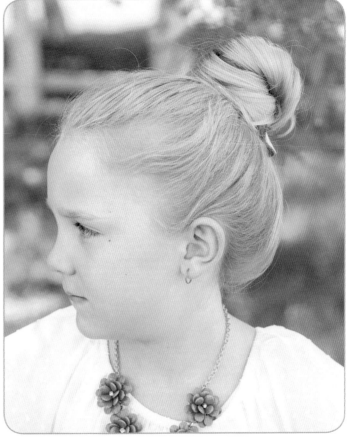

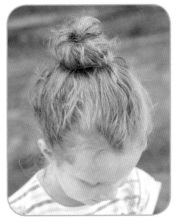

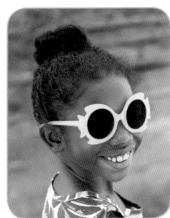

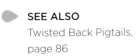
SEE ALSO
Twisted Back Pigtails, page 86

Get the look

WHAT YOU NEED

- Brush or comb
- Hair elastic
- Bobby pins
- Medium-hold hairspray

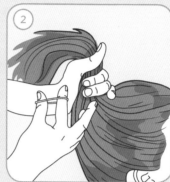

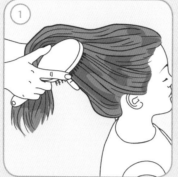

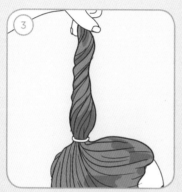

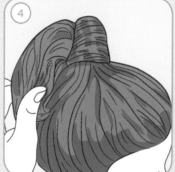

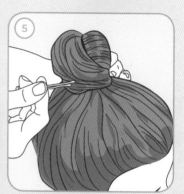

1. Brush or comb the hair until it is smooth and free from tangles. Gather into a high ponytail.

2. Secure the ponytail in place with an elastic.

3. Hold the ponytail straight up in the air and begin twisting.

4. As you twist, form a bun around the elastic at the base of the ponytail.

5. Pin in place with bobby pins. Spritz with hairspray to hold the twisty bun in place all day.

TOP TIP

This look works best with thick hair. If the hair is a little fine, then do two twists to make it look fuller.

Messy Top Knot

The messy top knot is the number-one hairdo for mums on the go. While it appears undone, it's cleverly crafted and requires a little more than throwing your bedhead hair into a knot. This look is great for mid- to long-length hair with medium to thick hair texture. Since wavy to curly hair already has the fullness required naturally, you can create this bun with minimum effort. With its messy nature, this top bun is suited to a playdate, park fun or a fun get-together with friends.

DIFFICULTY LEVEL
Easy

IDEAL HAIR
Medium to long; wavy to curly

ACCESSORIES
Add a pop of colour to this style with a headband.

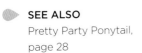 **SEE ALSO**
Pretty Party Ponytail, page 28

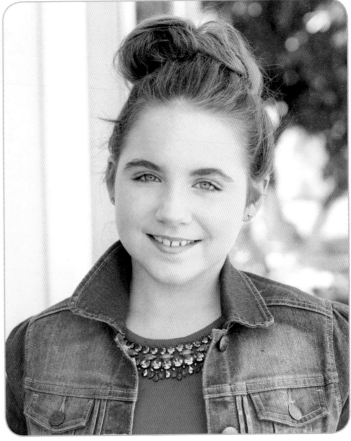

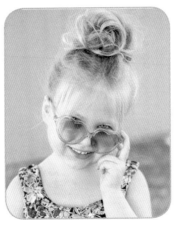

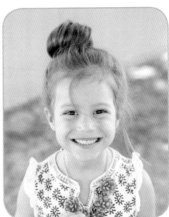

Get the look

WHAT YOU NEED

- Brush or comb
- Hair elastic
- Bobby pins
- Medium-hold hairspray

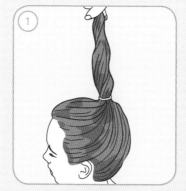

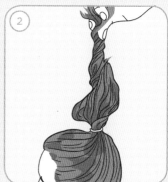

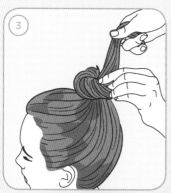

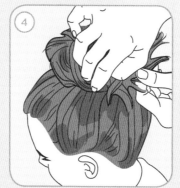

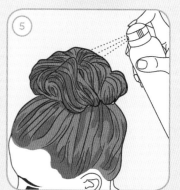

1. Brush or comb the hair until it is smooth and free from tangles. Gather into a high ponytail and secure in place with an elastic. Take the ponytail and pull it straight up from the elastic.

2. Slightly tease the hair, pulling straight down the strands of hair from the tip of the ponytail to the elastic with your fingers, while holding onto the tip of the ponytail.

3. Take the teased hair and loosely wrap it around the elastic at the base of the ponytail.

4. Secure the bun in place with bobby pins.

5. Mist with hairspray to set.

TOP TIP

This style works best when the hair has texture. Create on hair that has been washed the day before or add some dry shampoo.

Twisty Messy Low Bun

This is one of the best hairdos for when you're short on time. It's super quick, super simple and super pretty. It is great for hair that has texture from curly to wavy, ideally on mid to long lengths. It's the best for flyaways too because it adds to the messiness. While it's a casual look, paired with the right outfit, this bun can easily be dressed up for a more formal event.

DIFFICULTY LEVEL
Easy

IDEAL HAIR
Medium to long; fine to medium texture; wavy to curly

ACCESSORIES
Glam it up with some special accessories like pearls or diamanté studs in and around the bun.

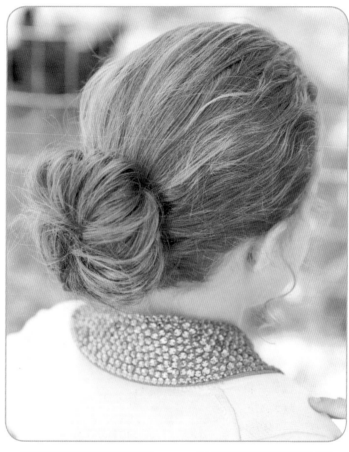

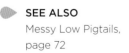 **SEE ALSO**
Messy Low Pigtails, page 72

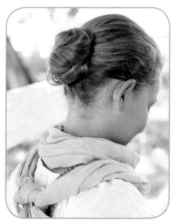

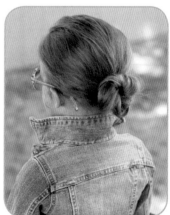

Get the look

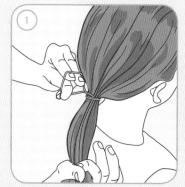

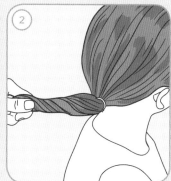

WHAT YOU NEED

- Brush or comb
- Hair elastic
- Bobby pins
- Medium-hold hairspray

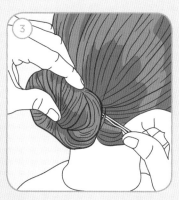

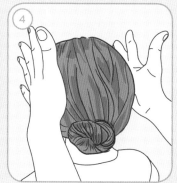

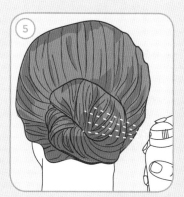

1. Brush or comb the hair until it is smooth and free from tangles. Gather the hair into a low ponytail and secure in place with an elastic.

2. Hold the hair from the ponytail straight out from the head and twist.

3. Wrap the twisted ponytail around the elastic at the base, pinning it in place with bobby pins.

4. Create a messy texture by rubbing your palms against the hair.

5. Spritz with hairspray to finish the bun and set the look.

TOP TIP

If the hair is fine, create a fuller bun by finger teasing the hair before you start. It will be fuller and create a messier look.

Formal Curly Bun

Can you believe this glam bun was created from a casual high ponytail? Whether your child has straight hair, curly hair or a mixture of both, this is the perfect low-maintenance style that not only looks pretty but keeps the hair out of their face too. This playful updo is also one of the best for thin hair because it adds instant volume.

DIFFICULTY LEVEL
Easy

IDEAL HAIR
Medium; medium to thick texture

ACCESSORIES
You can take this look to another level using diamantés, glitter hairspray or pearl hair accessories dotted throughout.

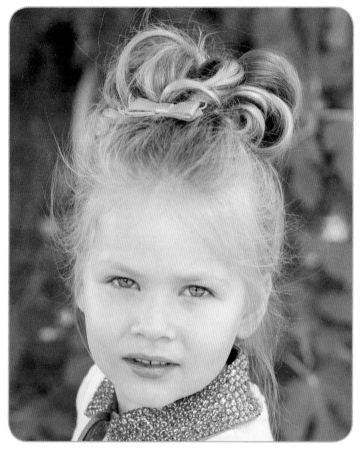

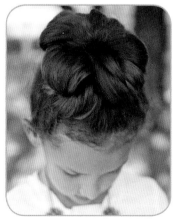

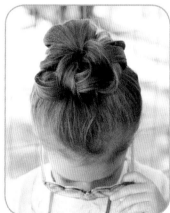

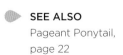 **SEE ALSO**
Pageant Ponytail, page 22

Get the look

WHAT YOU NEED

- Brush or comb
- Hair elastic
- 2.5-cm (1-inch) curling tongs
- Bobby pins
- Medium-hold hairspray

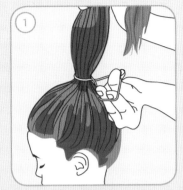

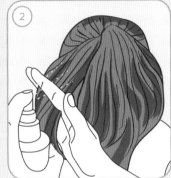

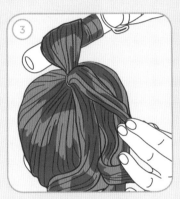

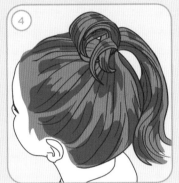

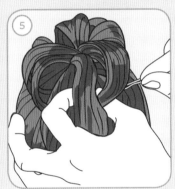

1. Brush or comb the hair until it is smooth and free from tangles. Gather the hair into a high ponytail and secure in place with an elastic.
2. Separate the ponytail into 1.2-cm (½-inch) sections and spritz each one with hairspray.
3. Curl a section of hair. Secure the curl in place with a bobby pin around the elastic.
4. Repeat step 3 until you run out of hair inside the ponytail.
5. Finish the look with some medium-hold hairspray all over the bun to keep it in place and minimise flyaways.

TOP TIP

If the hair is fine, lightly tease each section after curling, before pinning into place. If the hair is thick, wrap the curls tightly before pinning to reduce length and thickness.

Flower Bun

Taking inspiration from nature, this stunning style turns a simple braid into a delicate flower bun. Once you've mastered the look, you could up the style stakes by adding some real flowers to the finished bun. Small, delicate daisies or miniature roses would work best. This hairstyle works for dance recitals and most formal occasions, including weddings.

DIFFICULTY LEVEL
Medium

IDEAL HAIR
Long; medium to thick; straight to wavy

ACCESSORIES
Use a headband to set the look, or add some sparkle with glitter spray.

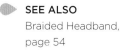 **SEE ALSO**
Braided Headband, page 54

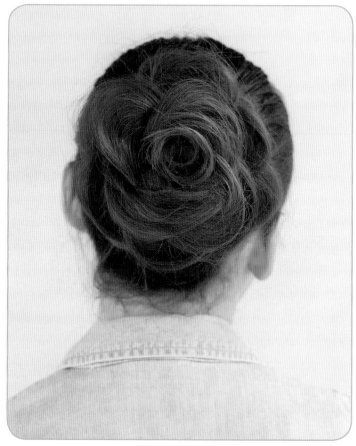

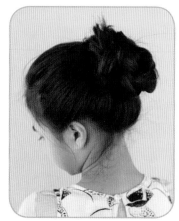 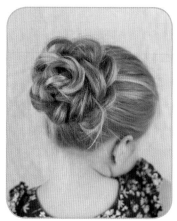

Get the look

WHAT YOU NEED

- Brush or comb
- Hair elastics
- Hair clip
- Bobby pins

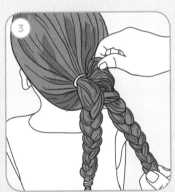
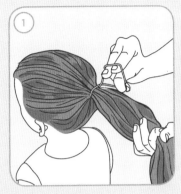
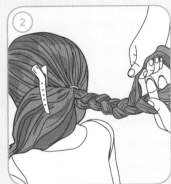
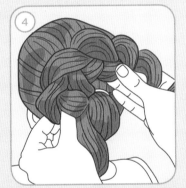
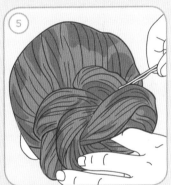

1. Brush or comb the hair until it is smooth and free from tangles. Gather the hair into a ponytail at the back of the head and secure in place with an elastic.

2. Divide the ponytail into two equal sections. Use the three-strand braiding technique (see page 25) to braid each section.

3. Use your fingers to stretch the outer side of each braid.

4. Wrap the left braid around the base of the ponytail tightly, placing the side of the braid that was not stretched out against the elastic. Pin it into place at the base of the braids.

5. Wrap the right braid in the same direction around the outside of your first flower braid, creating an outside layer of your flower bun. Secure in place with bobby pins.

TOP TIP

If the hair is straight and has a lot of layers, add a tiny bit of curl to the hair before beginning the braid. The curl will help the hair to blend into the braid and not stick out.

Minnie Mouse Ear Buns

This look is a must for all the Disney fans. Who needs to buy the theme park's classic mouse ears when you can recreate them with your child's hair? Your child will love this playful style, and your friends will be all ears when you tell them how simple it is. While it's a great option for birthday parties and Halloween, we love this fun updo for school too.

DIFFICULTY LEVEL
Medium

IDEAL HAIR
Medium to long; thick texture; wavy to frizzy

ACCESSORIES
Complete the Minnie Mouse look with a mini bow and a headband.

 SEE ALSO
Elsa Braid,
page 66

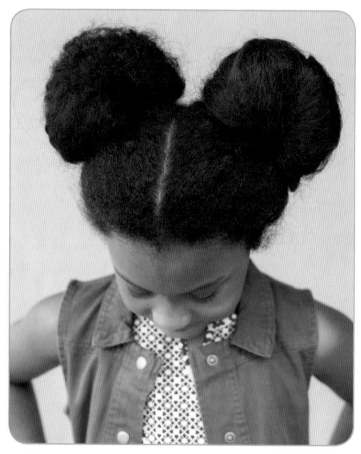

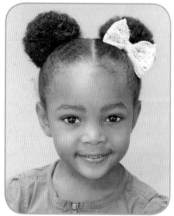

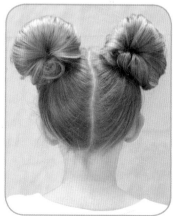

Get the look

WHAT YOU NEED

- Brush or comb
- Hair elastics
- Bobby pins

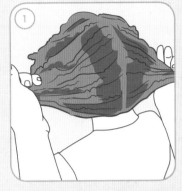

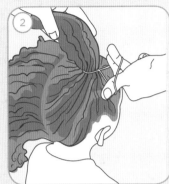

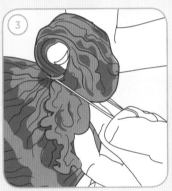

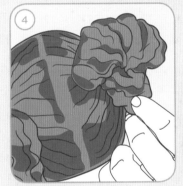

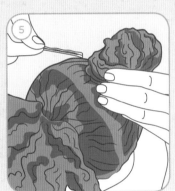

1. Brush or comb the hair until it is smooth and free from tangles. Make a centre parting.

2. Gather the hair into a ponytail on each side, 5 to 7.5 cm (2 to 3 inches) above the ear. Secure in place with elastics.

3. Pull one loop of the elastic out from where it is securing the ponytail and make a loop of hair over your thumb. Tuck the end of the ponytail through the loop. Secure the loop of hair in place with another elastic.

4. Spread out the hair in your loop to make a U-shape.

5. Tuck the ends up into your ear bun, securing in place with a bobby pin. Repeat on the other side.

TOP TIP

This hairstyle works beautifully on thick hair. For thin hair, create fullness by teasing the hair inside the ponytail before creating the ears.

Bow Bun

If you're looking for a fun twist on the traditional bun styles, this adorable bow bun is for you. It's a way of tying up short hair, making it ideal for those difficult in-between hair lengths when growing it out. This chic bun looks tricky to do but it's actually easy. Because it looks so playful, it's a great hairstyle for themed parties or playdates and can be dressed up with a cute bow for formal occasions.

DIFFICULTY LEVEL
Easy

IDEAL HAIR
Long; thick texture; straight or curly

ACCESSORIES
Use a mini bow or stylish hair clip and fix it to the top of the bun for added cuteness.

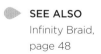 **SEE ALSO**
Infinity Braid, page 48

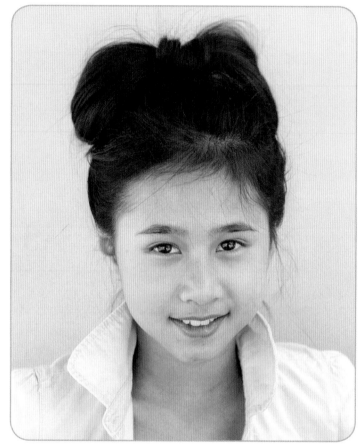

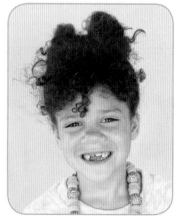

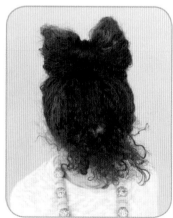

Get the look

WHAT YOU NEED
- Brush or comb
- Hair elastics
- Bobby pins

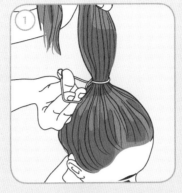

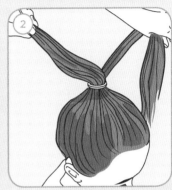

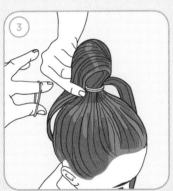

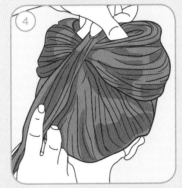

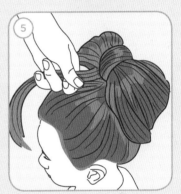

1. Brush or comb the hair until it is smooth and free from tangles. Gather the hair into a ponytail at the top of the head. Secure in place with an elastic.

2. Inside your ponytail, section out a 2.5- to 5-cm (1- to 2-inch) piece of hair and put it to one side.

3. Take the rest of the hair inside your ponytail and bend it in half to make a loop. Secure the loop in place with an elastic.

4. Split your loop in half. Take the small section that you put to one side and drape it over the middle of your loop to create your 'bow'.

5. Take the leftover ends from the section of hair that was draped over and bobby pin into place, moving it forwards and backwards around the centre of the bow until all of the hair is tucked away.

TOP TIP

If the hair is silky, add some light hair mist to the hair prior to folding in half. This will give silky hair some much-needed texture so it's easier to work with.

Ballerina Bun

While it might look pretty and polished, the ballerina bun is strong and durable – after all, it was created to survive a stage performance. While it will take some time to perfect the look, once you nail the basics, it's fairly simple. If you are creating this look for a recital, then get some practice and give your child a ballerina bun for playdates. When it is time for your child's performance, you'll be a pro.

DIFFICULTY LEVEL
Medium

IDEAL HAIR
Long; medium to thick; straight or wavy

ACCESSORIES
Fix a sweet hair bow or fun clip to the top.

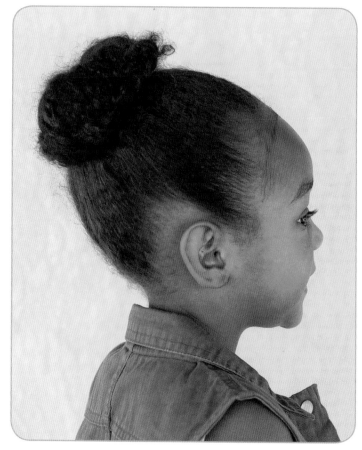

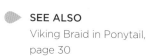 **SEE ALSO**
Viking Braid in Ponytail, page 30

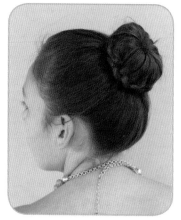

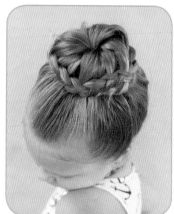

Get the look

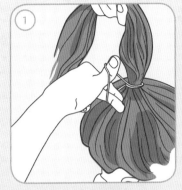

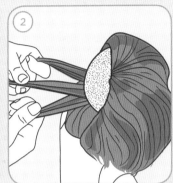

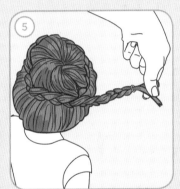

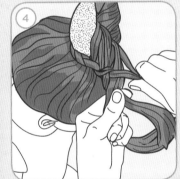

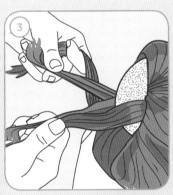

1. Brush or comb the hair until it is smooth and free from tangles. Gather the hair into a high ponytail. Secure with an elastic.

2. Divide a small section of hair from the underside of the ponytail. Thread the larger section of the ponytail through the doughnut. Divide the small section of hair into three.

3. Begin a three-strand braid (see page 25), working right then left. Braid three times, then start adding hair into the braid from the ponytail inside the doughnut. Add the hair to the right side of the braid only.

4. As you braid, direct the hair to form a circle covering the doughnut, forming the bun, then braid to the ends. Secure with an elastic.

5. Wrap the braid around the bun, securing in place with bobby pins and tucking the end of the braid underneath the bun.

TOP TIP

This style looks best if created in clean sections. Add a smoothing cream to the hair prior to styling to ensure your hair sections will be easy to work with.

Heart-shaped Bun

Turn the love dial up with this adorable heart-shaped bun. While this cute and creative take on the typical bun style looks like it would be difficult, it's actually easy. This chic classic is an obvious choice for formal affairs and a lovely look for parties, concerts and fun functions with friends.

DIFFICULTY LEVEL
Easy

IDEAL HAIR
Long; straight to wavy texture; minimal layers

ACCESSORIES
A hair bow is the perfect accent to finish the look.

 SEE ALSO
Heart Braid,
page 68

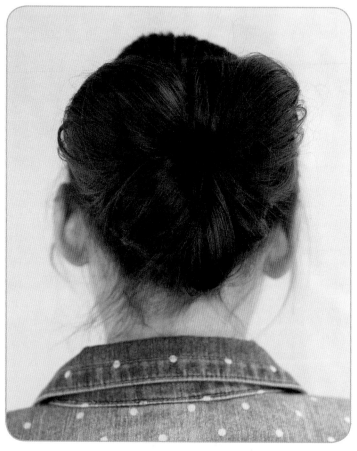

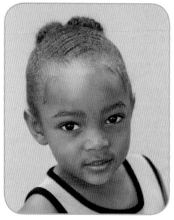

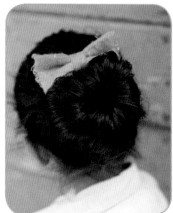

Get the look

WHAT YOU NEED
- Sock-bun doughnut
- Hair elastics
- Brush or comb
- Bobby pins

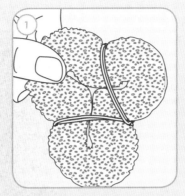

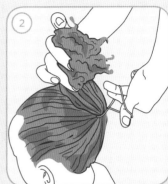

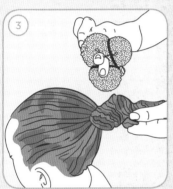

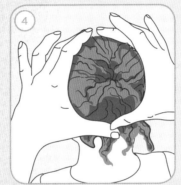

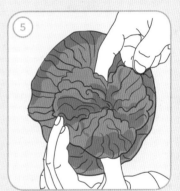

1. Add an elastic around all sides of the sock-bun doughnut to create a 'heart' shape.

2. Brush or comb the hair until it is smooth and free from tangles. Gather the hair into a ponytail at the back of the head and secure in place with an elastic.

3. Open the middle of your doughnut with your fingers and pull the ponytail through it.

4. Evenly spread all the hair out and around your heart-shaped doughnut. Take the ends of the hair, twist them around the doughnut and secure them in place with bobby pins.

5. Make your heart shape more defined by pushing in the indent in the heart shape and placing bobby pins into the bun to create definition.

TOP TIP

Create a larger heart shape by using a larger sock-bun doughnut. Secure an elastic on each side of your doughnut and then follow the tutorial to make your shape.

Cinderella Bun

Recreate Cinderella's stunning look at the ball on your own little princess. This elegant updo is perfect for formal occasions. Add a pretty headband to mimic the classic movie style for a themed birthday party, fun dress-up day, dance lesson, school or Halloween. It's mum and kid approved because it's cute and quick.

DIFFICULTY LEVEL
Hard

IDEAL HAIR
Medium to long; thick texture; silky

ACCESSORIES
Tie a pretty hair ribbon at the crown, or add a sweet blue headband to get the Cinderella look at the ball.

 SEE ALSO
Elsa Braid,
page 66

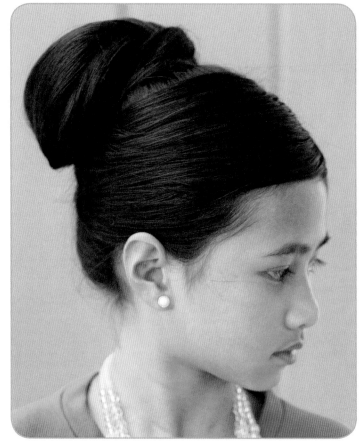

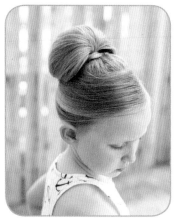

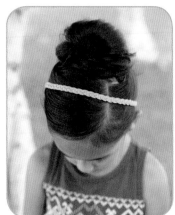

Get the look

WHAT YOU NEED

- Brush or comb
- Hair elastic
- Hair clip
- Bobby pins

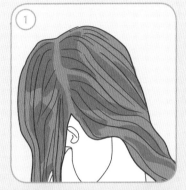

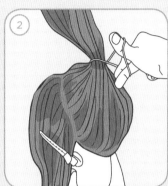

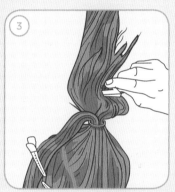

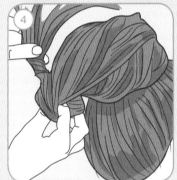

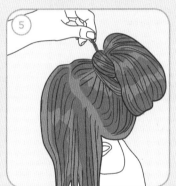

1. Brush the hair, making a deep side parting on the left. Section the hair at the front from the ears to the forehead, and clip.

2. Gather the unclipped hair into a high ponytail. Secure in place with an elastic.

3. Split the ponytail in half and clip the front away. Tease sections of the ponytail at the roots. Form the teased section into a large full bun. Secure in place with bobby pins.

4. Unclip the other half of the ponytail and drape it over the teased bun. Twist the ends of the hair and tuck underneath the bun.

5. Secure the bun with bobby pins and unclip the front section. Following the side parting, drape the hair around the back of the head, underneath the bun and then over around the base of the bun. Pin into place.

TOP TIP

If the hair is curly or frizzy, apply a smoothing lotion and blow dry with a large round brush before you begin. This will create a sleek finish.

Braided Bun

This is a classic look on a simple bun. It doesn't take long to style and you can create it on wet or dry hair, making it a quick and easy updo during the morning rush. It can be dressed up or down depending on the occasion. If you want to style this for a wedding, add some cute accessories or clips to create a formal-inspired look.

DIFFICULTY LEVEL
Medium

IDEAL HAIR
Long; medium texture; wavy or straight

ACCESSORIES
Style with a sweet bow or a fun headband.

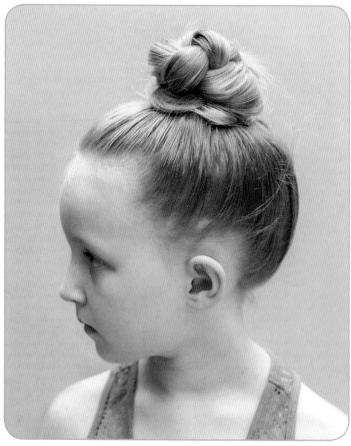

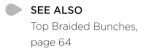 **SEE ALSO**
Top Braided Bunches, page 64

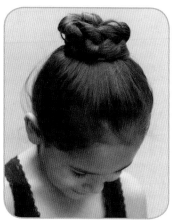

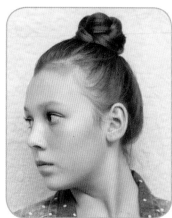

Get the look

WHAT YOU NEED

- Brush or comb
- Hair elastics
- Bobby pins

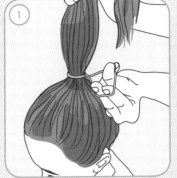

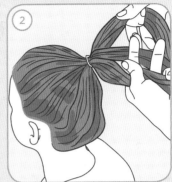

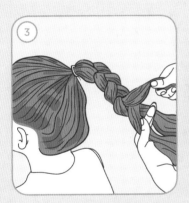

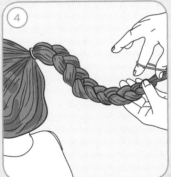

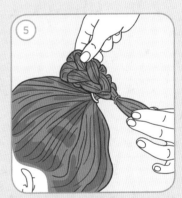

1. Brush or comb the hair until it is smooth and free from tangles. Gather the hair into a high ponytail and secure in place with an elastic.

2. Divide the hair inside the ponytail into three sections.

3. Begin to braid using the simple three-strand braid technique (see page 25), working right then left.

4. Continue to braid until you reach the ends of the hair. Secure in place with an elastic.

5. Take the braid and wrap it around the hair elastic at the top of the head to create the bun. Secure in place with bobby pins.

TOP TIP

If the hair is fine, stretch the braid with your fingers to create fullness before wrapping it around the elastic to create a bigger braided bun.

Resources

FURTHER EDUCATION

Love styling hair and want to do it every day? You can create a career out of making people look and feel beautiful as a cosmetologist.

Hairdressing is a rewarding career that combines technical skills with a creative, communicative outlet, and offers flexibility and the opportunity to run your own freelance business or salon. You'll also be able find work almost anywhere in the world.

To be a successful hairdresser, you'll need to be a good communicator. Hairdressing is a very social career. When people go to the salon, it's not just their hair that's expecting attention; people go for an experience. You'll have to be a people person, love listening and be able to keep up with all your clients' lives.

It's important you understand colour, shape and style, and being able to visualise the end result is vital. Styling hair also requires an impressive number of skills in order to become proficient. Everyone's hair is different, so you'll need to be artistic and creative, with a flair for solving problems. On top of this you'll need to be interested in – and good at – following trends, and be on the lookout to start your own.

Most of all, you'll need to love hair, fashion and style. If you have all these qualities, you'll make one heck of a hair stylist! Good luck!

The licensing requirements to register as a cosmetologist or hairdresser vary by country, so it's best to find a school in your area. Here are some websites to follow up if you're interested in pursuing a career as a hairdresser.

Schools:

Sassoon Academy (UK, USA, CANADA AND GERMANY)
sassoon.com

London Hair Academy (UK)
thelondonhairacademy.com

Saks Academy (UK)
saks.co.uk

Love hair and just want to find out more ways to style yours or your child's? Head online to these sites to discover more about how to look after and style hair:

theconfessionsofahairstylist.com
hairromance.com
latest-hairstyles.com
cutegirlshairstyles.com
princesshairstyles.com
hdofblog.com
twistmepretty.com
hairandmakeupbysteph.com

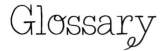

Glossary

Braid
Also referred to as a plait, a technique that involves weaving sections of hair into each other. There are several ways you can braid your hair, including three-strand braids, French braids and fishtail braids.

Crown
This is the area of the head along the top and back of the skull.

Curling tongs/wand
A round- or conical-barrel heat styling tool that creates curls and waves.

Dry shampoo
A hairstyling product that helps greasy or second-day hair look freshly washed. It's also a good product for adding texture to hair before styling.

Duck-bill clip
Long, slim clip used for holding the hair during styling.

French braid
The same as a French plait, see page 44.

Hair mist
Anti-frizz in a bottle: it makes dry hair soft and shiny.

Hair powder/micro dust
A light styling powder used at the roots to add volume and lift.

Hair section
A section of your hair that is clipped back while you work on other sections.

Hair texture
A term used to classify the type of hair you have depending on the curl pattern, volume and consistency of your hair.

Mousse
A light, fast-drying foam that gives extra volume, texture and shine. It can be used on wet or dry hair.

Nape
The area at the back of your neck.

Neckline
The neckline is part of the hairline, but specifically refers to the hair that begins at the back of the neck.

Rat tail comb
Also known as a weaving comb, this type of comb has a fine-toothed side and a narrow end made of plastic or metal. It is great for taking perfect sections and partings.

Salt spray
A product that pulls moisture and oils out of the hair, dries it and coarsens the texture.

Shine serum
A product to smooth the hair and enhance shine.

Shine spray
A spray for adding texture and shine to fine hair.

Tease
Also known as backcombing, ratting, matting or French lacing. This technique involves combing small sections of hair from the ends towards the scalp, creating a cushion or base for hairstyles that require volume.

Photo Credits

Unless otherwise stated, hairstyling is by Jenny Strebe and her hair team, and photography is by Sara Bishop Photography.

Page 7 Top left: Jocelyn Duran
Top right: Hayden Rae Burke
Bottom left: Jayden Polkus
Bottom right: Kendall Peck

Page 11 Jenna Theisen

Page 13 Olivia Tengberg

CHAPTER ONE

Page 16 Top: Nia James
Bottom left: Lauren Harper
Bottom right: Olivia Tengberg

Page 18 Top: Tiffany Xoumphon
Bottom left and right: Danica Duran

Page 20 Top and bottom left: Hayden Rae Burke
Bottom right: Htoorahmu Pee

Page 22 Top: Kendall Peck
Bottom left: Danica Duran
Bottom right: Audianna Smith

Page 24 Top: Kaelyn Walls
Bottom left: Lauren Harper
Bottom right: Olivia Canyon

Page 26 Top: Adelyn Manogue
Bottom left: Zara Malik
Bottom right: Jayden Polkus

Page 28 Top: Jayden Polkus
Bottom left: Kenna Lott
Bottom right: Tiffany Xoumphon

Page 30 Top: Olivia Tengberg
Bottom left: Lauren Harper
Bottom right: Magnolia Strebe

Page 32 Top and bottom right: Tiffany Xoumphon
Bottom left: Hayden Rae Burke

Page 34 Top: Kendall Peck
Bottom left: Eliana Brown
Bottom right: Jayden Polkus

Page 36 Top and bottom left: Kendall Peck
Bottom right: Tiffany Xoumphon

Page 38 Top: Kaelyn Walls
Bottom left: Olivia Tengberg
Bottom right: Olivia Canyon

Page 40 Top: Braily Skousen
Bottom left and right: Jenna Theisen

CHAPTER TWO

Page 44 Top and bottom left: Adelyn Manogue
Bottom right: Jayden Polkus

Page 46 Top: Olivia Canyon
Bottom left: Isabella Stewart
Bottom right: Kaelyn Walls

Page 48 Top: Tiffany Xoumphon
Bottom left: Jesikah Perez
Bottom right: Magnolia Strebe

Page 50 Top and bottom left: Hayden Rae Burke
Bottom right: Zara Malik

Page 52 Top: Olivia Tengberg,
Bottom left: Braily Skousen
Bottom right: Liv Kelly

Page 54 Top: Kendall Peck
Bottom left: Htoorahmu Pee
Bottom right: Zara Malik

Page 56 Top: Kaelyn Walls
Bottom left: Lauren Harper
Bottom right: Magnolia Strebe

Page 58 Top: Kendall Peck
Bottom left: Tiffany Xoumphon
Bottom right: Htoorahmu Pee

Page 60 Top and bottom right: Hayden Rae Burke
Bottom left: Tiffany Xoumphon

Page 62 Top: Olivia Tengberg
Bottom left: Isabella Stewart
Bottom right: Jenna Theisen

Page 64 Top: Htoorahmu Pee
Bottom left: Zara Malik
Bottom right: Audianna Smith

Page 66 Top: Isabella Stewart
Bottom left: Magnolia Strebe
Bottom right: Jenna Theisen

Page 68 Top: Kendall Peck
Bottom left: Jayden Polkus
Bottom right: Jesikah Perez

CHAPTER THREE

Page 72 Top: Nia James
Bottom left: Coco Bagley
Bottom right: Liv Kelly

Page 74 Top: Magnolia Strebe
Bottom left: Danica Duran
Bottom right: Adelyn Manogue

Page 76 Top: Braily Skousen
Bottom left: Adelynn Skousen
Bottom right: Jenna Theisen

Page 78 Top: Tiffany Xoumphon
Bottom left: Danica Duran
Bottom right: Magnolia Strebe

Page 80 Top: Eliana Brown
Bottom left: Hayden Rae Burke
Bottom right: Adelynn Skousen

Page 82 Top: Nia James
Bottom left: Liv Kelly
Bottom right: Coco Bagley

Page 84 Top: Jenna Theisen
Bottom left: Adelynn Skousen
Bottom right: Coco Bagley

Page 86 Top: Kendall Peck
Bottom left and right: Audianna Smith

Page 88 Top and bottom left: Kenna Lott
Bottom right: Adelynn Skousen

Page 90 Top: Isabella Stewart
Bottom left: Magnolia Strebe
Bottom right: Nia James

Page 92 Top: Hayden Rae Burke
Bottom left and right: Htoorahmu Pee

Page 94 Top: Magnolia Strebe
Bottom left: Liv Kelly
Bottom right: Jenna Theisen

CHAPTER FOUR

Page 98 Top: Kenna Lott
Bottom left: Danica Duran
Bottom right: Adelyn Manogue

Page 100 Top: Olivia Tengberg
Bottom left: Liv Kelly
Bottom right: Nia James

Contributors

HAIR

Head Hair Stylist
Jenny Strebe
theconfessionsofahairstylist.com

Hair Stylists
Demi Walsh
styleseat.com/theoryhairdesign

Anthony Lunam
styleseat.com/theoryhairdesign

Hair Assistants
Tanner Johnson
Emily Finn
Emily Armijo

PHOTOGRAPHY

Sara Bishop
sarabishop.com

Photography Assistant
Catolyn Lunt

Photo shoot location

Webster Farm
instagram.com/websterfarm

CLOTHING

Head Clothing Stylist
Reachel Bagley
cardiganempire.com

Assistant Clothing Stylist
Tiffany Cook
grownupdressup.com

Assistant Clothing Stylist
Celeste Chelsey

MODELS

Adelyn Manogue

Adelynn Skousen

Audianna Smith

Braily Skousen

Coco Bagley

Danica Duran

Eliana Brown

Hayden Rae Burke

Htoorahmu Pee

Isabella Stewart

Jayden Polkus

Jenna Theisen

Jesikah Perez

Jocelyn Duran

Kaelyn Walls

Kendall Peck

Kenna Lott

Lauren Harper

Liv Kelly

Magnolia Strebe

Nia James

Olivia Canyon

Olivia Tengberg

Tiffany Xoumphon

Zara Malik

Index

Acknowledgements

This book has been an absolute dream to work on thanks to my incredible support team who have so kindly donated their talents and time to making this book happen. The first of many thank yous has to go to my supportive husband, Casey, whose constant love, patience and encouragement has given me the strength to pursue my passion. You are my rock, thank you. To my kids, your unconditional love means everything to me and helps me face the many challenges along the way. Thank you for always being my number one fans. A massive thank you to my photographer, Sara Bishop, you are an absolute star and super talented woman. I'm so grateful to have you in my corner. Thank you Webster Farm for letting us use your beautiful location as our set for the photographs. To my champion hair assistants, Demi Walsh and Anothony Luam, thanks for being my expert wingmen. The shoots all ran so smoothly thanks to you both. To my brilliant editor, Erin, for your guidance and amazing organisational skills. We couldn't have kept to the deadlines without you, so thank you. And a massive thank you to my awesome ghost writer, Sacha Strebe, because I really could not have done this book without you.